Transforming Health and Beauty:

Red Light Therapy for You and Your Pets

Dr. Cie Allman-Scott

TRANSFORMING HEALTH AND BEAUTY: Red Light Therapy for You and Your Pets

For information address Dr. Cie Scott, 11201 N. Tatum Blvd., Suite 300, Phoenix, AZ 85028.

Dr. Cie Scott's books may be purchased for educational, business, or sales promotional use.

For information please write: Dr. Cie Scott, Special Markets Department, Infinite Power Media, 11201 N. Tatum Blvd., Suite 300, Phoenix, AZ 85028. TRANSFORMING HEALTH & BEAUTY: Red Light Therapy for You and Your Pets

FIRST EDITION

Allman-Scott, Cie.

Transforming Health & Beauty: Red Light Therapy for You and Your Pets

/Cie Allman-Scott.

ISBN 978-0-9774811-6-3

To my husband who has saved many lives as a surgeon and has thankfully experienced rapid and remarkable results from Red Light Therapy. I also dedicate this book to my dogs who trust and enjoy RLT every chance they get. I also deeply appreciate all who have taken the time to assist me and support my endeavors to facilitate happiness, cellular health, and fitness. We enthusiastically offer a better mind, body, and Spirit, and ultimately longevity to everyone. Whether you are already healthy and want to discover new modalities for anti-aging and health, or you desperately need it and are not yet informed, this is for you, your family, your pets, and everyone you care about.

Medical Disclaimer

The information in this book about red light therapy is provided solely for educational and informational purposes. This information does not replace professional medical advice, diagnosis, or treatment.

The publisher and author of this book have ensured that the information provided is accurate and up-to-date. However, the data may be incomplete or may become obsolete over time.

Before beginning any new therapy or treatment, including red light therapy, the reader should consult a qualified healthcare professional. This book should not be used to diagnose or treat medical conditions nor as a replacement for professional medical advice.

This book's author and publisher are not liable for any consequences or adverse effects that may result from its use or application. The reader undertakes full responsibility for his or her actions and decisions based on the contents of this book. Therefore, any dependence on such information is strictly at your discretion. In conclusion, readers of this book on red light therapy should always consult a qualified healthcare professional and use the information contained in this book at their peril. The author and publisher of this book disclaim any liability or responsibility for any adverse outcomes or consequences that may result from using or applying the information contained in this book.

Contents

Introduction

Every morning when I wake up at home, I get out of bed and before I get dressed or have my green, pre-breakfast drink, I lay down for a session in my red and infrared light therapy bed. The moment my dogs notice that I'm getting in, they jump out of bed and jump into the RLT bed with me. They must inherently know that it is good for them and that they have felt stronger and healthier since their sessions began. They refuse to be left out!

After many brief impressions, I eventually realized the incredible value of RLT first in Las Vegas at the American Academy of Anti-Aging Medicine (A4M) Conference in 2021. It finally had my full attention! Two months later, a dear friend in the medical field became the VP and Director at Cerulean Human Health Performance. She hired me to promote Cerulean and I suggested that we film a TV episode of *Beauty and Truth* at her world-class center. As you age, your telomeres get shorter. At Cerulean, they lengthen your telemeres and although they cannot chronologically change your age, they can make your cells “younger,” altering the way you perform and look. They have many wealthy clients who want to improve their energy, health and appearance, and professional athletes that depend on their modalities to help them recover from their sports and lengthen their professional careers. Other than being paid, the best benefit at Cerulean turned out to be VIP treatment and the ability to use the modalities myself. From the first time I used their RLT bed, I knew I had to own one. For maximum benefits, you cannot wear sunscreen, makeup or a stitch of clothing. Removing sunscreen is an extra step if you wear it religiously like I do.

I enjoyed my treatments at Cerulean and eventually asked where they acquired their bed. I found the owner of the company and asked him to have lunch with me. We got along famously and within a couple of months, I had one of these incredible anti-aging machines at a price I could afford. My husband, a General and Vascular Surgeon thought I was not aligned with my sensibilities when I paid for this bed, even though he didn't try to stop me. I urged him to use it; I am the picture of health but my husband has many physical issues; some are congenital and some he discovered in his thirties. After four days of using the bed his life changed. He could feel it and in utter surprise he admitted to me that his energy had changed. He could feel the systems of his body improve. The chronic pain in his back quickly became totally manageable to the point that he removed all of the old solar panels off the roof of our home in one day. The younger workers from a roofing company that witnessed this feat were in shock and awe. As all wives know, hearing the words, "You were right!" are rare, and more importantly it was a thrill to know this modality also worked miracles for him.

My household, medical and psychological by profession, includes my certified therapy dogs. We are fully committed to this amazing modality for longevity and health.

Chapter 1: History & Evolution Of RLT

"Future medicine will be the medicine of frequencies."

-Albert Einstein

Let there be light for your irritated skin, wounds, and other injuries. The use of red light as a potential treatment for various health and aesthetic issues is just beginning to gain traction due to the interest shown by researchers, universities, and hospitals. The availability of at-home equipment makes it more approachable.

Discover the background of the treatment, its mechanism of action, the possible benefits it may offer, what to anticipate throughout treatment, and more by reading on.

The Origins & Development of RLT

The use of red light therapy (RLT) as part of a day-to-day wellness regimen has grown significantly in popularity over the past several years. It has many applications, including treating skin conditions, managing chronic pain, promoting better sleep, anti-aging effects, and preventing hair loss, among a growing list. Later in this chapter, we explore some of the most important events that have occurred throughout the history of red light therapy. The practice of light treatment did not begin to change into what it is now until the discovery of wavelengths of light and the invention of optics.

Modern Optics & Photonics

Thomas Edison created the idea for the first functional electric light bulb in 1879. This innovation paved the way for light therapy, which had previously relied on natural light from the sun.

In 1893, Dr. Finsen, a Danish physician, introduced ultraviolet light therapy by utilizing artificial light sources instead of relying on the sun's natural light. This groundbreaking approach marked the first instance of employing isolated wavelengths of light for therapeutic purposes.

Dr. Finsen was suffering from a severe kind of neurodegenerative illness known as Pick's disease. He discovered that spending time in the sun reduced the severity of his ailments, and this launched his interest in the healing capabilities of light. He was successful in curing lupus vulgaris, which is a kind of tuberculosis.

In 1903, Dr. Finsen won a Nobel Prize in Medicine for using light therapy to heal tuberculosis (by applying ultraviolet light) and scars left by smallpox (by applying red light). These initial light treatments were laborious because Dr. Finsen could only treat a 2cm area at a time, and each treatment took several hours daily. Despite this limitation in size, the treatments were effective in removing the lesions. Finsen's results were well worth the effort.

History of Light Therapy

Heliotherapy refers to the practice of using natural sunlight for medical purposes. This practice has existed for centuries. The Greek word Helios, which translates as "Sun," is the origin of it. Artificial sources of ultraviolet, visible, or infrared radiation for therapeutic purposes are now included in Heliotherapy.

Sunlight therapy has been used worldwide for medical and psychiatric treatment by ancient healers who believed the sun could heal. People have been practicing sunlight therapy for thousands of years.

Isaac Newton's scientific studies with prisms and light in 1666, which led to breakthroughs in understanding the qualities of light, are credited with marking the so-called 'annus mirabilis' or marvelous year.

Newton conducted tests using sunlight and prisms, uncovering that clear white light consisted of seven discernible hues. These investigations led to the discovery of the light spectrum. His work from 1666 laid the groundwork for his second masterwork book, which he published in 1704 regarding optics.

Experiments Conducted By NASA

NASA was interested in establishing the capability to cultivate plants in space to reshape the future of interplanetary exploration. They tried out this theory by growing food indoors as an experiment.

The purpose of the red light experiment conducted by NASA was to determine whether or not red wavelengths of visible light may encourage plant growth aboard spacecraft. Using traditional grow lights aboard spacecraft is challenging because of the high amount of electricity they consume and the heat they produce.

Research has demonstrated that red light-emitting diodes (LEDs) provide helpful illumination for plants because of their compact size, risk-free operation, and low level of wasted heat.

The researchers who were responsible for cultivating these plants were also exposed to red light, leading to their hands healing rapidly and unexpectedly. This was referred to as the "happy accident."

Subsequent research into the effects of red light on human health was conducted almost immediately. The experiments employed both red and near-infrared (NIR) light. Red light therapy is an umbrella phrase that can refer to red light with wavelengths between 630 and 680 nanometers, near-infrared light with wavelengths between 800 and 1100 nanometers, or even a combination of the two.

Astronauts experience severe and potentially dangerous bone and muscle loss and a slowing of the healing process due to their zero-gravity environment. These issues arise from improper cell proliferation under zero-gravity conditions in spacecraft. This curiosity has sparked a desire to explore the effects of red light on the human body.

One of the earliest uses of red light therapy was to combat the adverse effects of zero-gravity conditions on the proliferation of individual cells. Researchers discovered that red light stimulates the metabolism of cellular material, enabling astronauts to maintain their muscle mass and bone density while in space. The revolutionary finding led to the establishment of red light therapy.

Red light has also found application as “grow lights” in horticulture on Earth. In the 1990s, there was a budding interest in red and near-infrared light as the 'therapeutic window' of visible and invisible light due to their numerous health benefits. This interest stemmed from discovering that red and near-infrared light is the only wavelength range within the visible and invisible light spectrum with healing properties.

Recent Scientific Developments

In the 20th century, we have witnessed a surge in interest in using light therapy across various medical specialties, including dermatology, cardiology, and ophthalmology.

Albert Einstein developed the concept of LASER (Light Amplification by Stimulated Emission of Radiation) in 1917. Despite the concept origins, the development of the technology did not really begin until the year 1960.

In the 1920s and 1930s, researchers realized that vitamin D was necessary for maintaining a healthy body and that exposure to sunlight prompted the body to produce more vitamin D. The use of ultraviolet light proved very effective in accomplishing this goal.

Even short skin exposure to UV rays could cause desirable changes in the body; this led to the widespread adoption of light treatment in the 20th century. 'Sun lamps' emitting ultraviolet (UV) rays were utilized to treat emotional disorders and various medical conditions, including rickets, psoriasis, lupus, fungal infections, eczema, and vitiligo.

During the 1950s, medical practitioners frequently used ultraviolet B (UVB) light to treat various dermatological diseases. The discovery that UVB light effectively treats hyperbilirubinemia, commonly known as neonatal jaundice, led to a significant increase in the utilization of UVB light.

A nurse at Rochford General Hospital in Essex, England discovered that sun exposure in specific areas reduced the symptoms of a jaundiced child. Dr. Dobbs, the attending physician, agreed that exposure to direct sunlight helped to resolve jaundice, confirming the nurse's discovery.

Phototherapy, often known as the therapeutic use of light, is still used to treat high bilirubin levels in neonates, even in today's modern medical world.

Modern photobiomodulation treatments for jaundice replace the previous use of ultraviolet light by utilizing light wavelengths ranging from 310 to 490 nanometers (nm).

Advancement in Light-Emitting Diode

In 1961, Robert Biard and Gary Pittman invented the light-emitting diode (LED). The small size of the early LEDs made them somewhat cumbersome and limited their usefulness.

Nick Holonyak, Jr., a scientist working for General Electric, is credited with inventing the first commercially viable and operational LED in 1962. He has now earned the title of the "Father of the Light Emitting Diode." LEDs were initially used as lights for circuit boards and other small electrical devices because they offered an alternative that was far more energy efficient than incandescent light bulbs. Since LEDs are much more energy efficient than halogen and incandescent lights, they are becoming increasingly commonplace in the lighting industry.

First and foremost, light-emitting diodes, or LEDs, can only create a single wavelength of light instead of the various wavelengths that incandescent light bulbs produce. Initially, they could only generate red wavelengths, but as time passed, they were improved to generate any wavelength of light imaginable.

LED light therapy devices designed for consumers today commonly emit blue, amber, red, and near-infrared light. Sometimes these colors are used singly, and sometimes they are used together. Research into colors of light other than blue or red, intending to develop different therapies, has been unsuccessful for the most part.

LED technology advanced significantly in the 1990s due to manufacturing innovations that made it less expensive and more efficient. The fact that it could deliver uniform wavelengths, just like lasers (although not to the same degree), was highly crucial to the medical field. LED devices have successfully recreated the effects shown in red light research conducted with lasers.

Compared to lasers, the primary advantage of contemporary LED light therapy devices is their capacity to transmit particular wavelengths of red and near-infrared light to a broader portion of the body. This convenience makes LED light therapy more suitable for treating large-scale illnesses like psoriasis and promoting overall health and wellness.

With the explosion of research into this natural treatment, the application of red light therapy has spread into many different areas, including the management of chronic pain, supportive care of cancer patients, treatment of neurological diseases, treatment of traumatic brain injury, oral mucositis, chronic skin conditions, and a great deal more. It has even become popular for hair restoration!

RLT Research

Gaining a more in-depth understanding of the mechanisms of action, particularly in inflammation, is of utmost importance as it is considered the underlying cause of many diseases. A 2017 study demonstrated the ability of red light therapy to reduce inflammation, 'shedding light' on why it is an immensely effective treatment for inflammatory arthritis.

In recent years, red light therapy has emerged as a powerful treatment for various medical and psychological ailments. It has become one of the most talked about topics in contemporary medicine.

Since the early 1990s, Dr. Michael Hamblin has been researching RLT as a potential treatment for various conditions, including wounds, traumatic brain injuries, arthritis, and hair regrowth. He has published nearly 300 papers based on his study findings.

In a March 2020 interview, Hamblin talked about using red light therapy and how he incorporates it into his routine. He stated that he consistently utilizes the method to alleviate soreness in his knees and elbows. He applies RLT to his forehead twice a week to enhance the overall health of his brain. According to Hamblin, red light treatment has demonstrated an anti-inflammatory effect in individuals suffering from chronic inflammation.

RLT has been shown in several trials to hasten the healing process. Furthermore, RLT exhibits a powerful curative impact, particularly beneficial in cases where underlying inflammation causes autoimmune diseases or other conditions.

Engineer and physicist Theodore H. Malman developed the first laser in 1960, receiving widely publicized credit for this achievement. A laser emits amplified light with a constant wavelength, allowing it to focus on a narrow beam.

Hungarian medical doctor, Endre Mester invented the first low-level laser therapy medical device in 1967. It was designed to treat skin cancer, delivering concentrated red and near-infrared light. In subsequent years, the device found application in accelerating wound healing.

Laser therapy finds applications in various medical specialties, such as dermatology and surgery, depending on the strength of the laser used. Low-level laser therapy is employed just like LED light therapy, to improve the vitality of cells, whereas more powerful "hot" lasers eliminate damaged and dead cells by vaporizing them.

Lasers are now commonly used in various fields, including the entertainment industry, catering to consumers. They are also valuable for various industrial and clinical settings, as we've discussed.

User-Friendly Aspects of RLT

It is now possible for everyone to reap the benefits of red-light treatment in the comfort of their own home due to the introduction of a growing number of high-quality medical-grade devices including the BIOMAX line from Platinum LED Treatment Lights.

Do LEDs have the same level of efficiency as lasers? According to the findings of a study that compared the effects of lasers and LEDs on the healing of wounds, the biological effects and characteristics of both types of light sources are relatively comparable. They result in a reduction of inflammation, an increase in collagen synthesis, and other beneficial healing effects.

Dangers Associated with RLT

The PBM (PhotoBioModulation) Foundation collaborates with senior science and government officials for improving acceptance and application of RLT. This foundation conducts research, educates and certifies and ultimately promotes PBM. This includes funding research and expanding insurance coverage. The Food and Drug Administration (FDA) in the United States of America has generally cleared red light therapy. Approval only comes with clinical data, and with over 100,000 various units available to the market, obviously most have not specifically been registered, cleared or approved. Even though red light therapy has been found to be safe, users can still make errors when using it in their homes. Using the gadget excessively or more frequently than the manufacturer indicates is possible. The good news is that many gadgets used at home come equipped with an automatic timer and shutoff feature, which makes it much simpler to avoid over-treatment. Always follow the recommendations because RLT could, for example, worsen some migraine symptoms.

Potential Advantages of RLT

There are still contradicting theories on red light treatment; some of these theories reveal no effect on health disorders but naturally studies also reveal success. Generally, there is a need for more standardization in studies across the board (in dosage and timing) depending on the disease or application, so medical professionals can completely comprehend the breadth of benefits that red light therapy can provide. The following is a list of possible promising applications for red light treatment, as determined by various experts; it is not in any particular order:

Youthful Skin

One frequently mentioned advantage of red light therapy is its ability to affect the skin in a positive way, and there are many applications that have been successful. Red light therapy can treat acne, fine lines and wrinkles, promote hair growth, reduce skin redness, and much more.

Dose Response Curve for Skin or Surface Issues

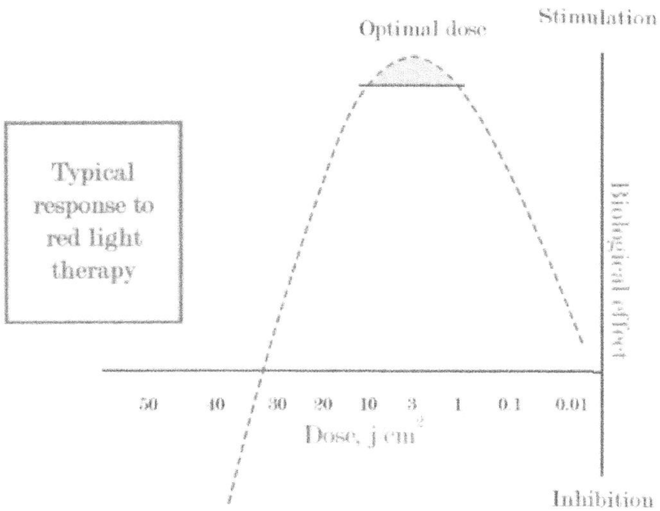

Red light therapy is known to reduce inflammation, which is beneficial in promoting healthy skin. Clearing up redness, acne, and skin ailments can aid topical or oral therapies for these and other conditions, allowing them to operate even more effectively. Red Light Therapy (RLT) also increases our immune defenses significantly against the bacteria associated with the formation of acne; this is an essential factor in inhibiting acne breakouts. These therapies target enzymes related to the breakdown of collagen and encourage the creation of collagen; this helps lessen the appearance of wrinkles and fine lines.

Rehabilitation of Sports Injuries

Red light treatment could help athletes recover after an injury that has rendered them immobile and incapacitated; the benefits may include both mental and physical improvements, which obviously would improve mood. Quoting Professor Praveen Arany, "Red light can be used to improve the performance of skeletal muscles, reduce pain, and improve recovery from injury." PBM has the potential to be employed both in the rehabilitation of sports injuries, and to increase athletic performance.

Healing Wounds

RLT expert and professor, Praveen Arany wrote a review on RLT's effect on wound healing. He was published in April 2019 in *Advances in Skin and Wound Care*. He explained "The anti-inflammatory characteristics of red light have been found to boost the body's ability to heal; this is true whether you have an open sore on your foot or an ulcer in your mouth."

Pain Management

Red light therapy has shown clinical results and promise as a potential method for alleviating pain, which is notoriously difficult to treat without drugs. Ph.D. and Doctor of Dental Sciences, Praveen Arany says, "Red light affects the neurons responsible for the transmission of pain."

Red light therapy may be more effective for certain kinds of pain than others. Red light may effectively treat painful illnesses such as fibromyalgia, osteoarthritis, neuropathy, and chronic low blood pressure.

Who Should Consider RLT

Red light therapy was originally intended to complement other treatments rather than serve as the sole treatment for health or skincare issues. To most, it is improbable for red light therapy to address their needs alone, but this mindset is changing. For example, to address concerns such as acne or fine wrinkles, you may also consider using a topical treatment like a retinoid in addition to RLT. Topical cream plus RLT studies are currently under way at Theralight, a prolific RLT manufacturer.

Healthy people like me can sometimes do daily treatments or treat 3 times a week as a total health regimen. I can feel improvement in ways I didn't expect in many systems of the body. It's not unusual to see measurable results in a short time (a few days).

Professor Praveen Arany advises pregnant women to avoid undergoing red light treatment. If you are seeking treatment for a specific medical issue, obtaining permission from your primary care physician is also suggested. In a 2023 discussion I had with Arany, he told me that women often have pain in their shoulders, neck and back, as well as edema in their feet during their pregnancy. He said that RLT is appropriate to relieve these issues, but he mentioned that focusing the light on the fetus is to be avoided. In other words, some sites are acceptable but systemic and full body beds are not a good idea during the pregnancy.

RLT Availability for the Consumer Market

PlatinumLED conducted the research and development necessary to create the industry's first 12-wave spectrum for horticulture use in 2012. These high-powered LEDs quickly became the grow-light standard in the horticulture industry worldwide.

In 2015, there was a transition from animal therapy to human therapy, and PlatinumLED was the first company to offer a high-powered LED panel with red and near-infrared options. At last, red light therapy was made available to the general public. I will share far more about the market, efficacy, applicability and how to find such devices for treatment later in this book.

Beginning the Process of RLT

Before you first try red light treatment under supervision or instruction, there are several things you must be aware of, as outlined in this chapter.

In most cases, RLT requires scheduling several appointments over a specific period of time. For skin issues, individuals should undergo red light therapy three times per week for at least one month, with each session lasting ten to thirty minutes. Protocols rely on the light, power and intensity. While some patients may notice results within a week, it is typical for the outcomes to improve gradually over time.

Before attempting red light treatment on your own, it is recommended to consult with a dermatologist or a pain specialist. An experienced medical professional helps establish your wellness goals, and may better determine if RLT suits you, regarding any medical conditions you might have, and may perhaps assist you in finding the specific at-home device worth investing your money.

The Science behind RLT

The use of light at particular wavelengths is at the heart of photobiomodulation; this is anywhere from 400 nanometers (nm) (blue) up to 1,100 nm (near infrared). This includes a great deal of 'light' energy that is not visible to humans. On the other hand, the National Centre for Atmospheric Research considers the wave lengths for red light to range from 630 to 680 nm. By that more narrow definition, Red light falls within the visible spectrum of light.

All three primary light colors, i.e., blue, green, and red, have been utilized successfully as PBM treatments. In addition to red light, Photobiomodulation (PBM) uses near-infrared light, which has a longer wavelength than visible light (up to 1,200 nm). Actually, infrared light warms the body but is not visible to the human eye. Many wavelengths of energy are not visible to humans, so infrared light is not unique in being invisible.

In recent years, red light therapy has grown in popularity and it is finally an easy-to-acquire treatment. It is now even offered in many medical and chiropractic offices, as well as health clubs and spas.

When photons, which are measures of light energy 'particles', are brought close to the skin, they penetrate and activate chromophores, which are components of molecules responsible for the color of that molecule; this absorption causes changes within cells. Red light treatment affects the mitochondria in cells. Mitochondria are considered the "powerhouses" of cells; this causes the production of ATP (the biological currency of energy), which helps the body function. This form of energy stimulation enhances the cell's ability to repair itself.

As you embark on RLT, the presence of a knowledgeable practitioner is helpful for the success of your treatment. This therapy involves specific protocols and dosages customized to each patient's unique health condition. If you are hesitant, try to receive this treatment in a clinical setting with trained medical personnel. Surprisingly, aesthetic practices or salons are doing well for most people to see the benefits of this treatment. Centers for athletic recovery are popping up in many cities where professional athletes play and train. Salons and spas are fine for seeking treatment for most healthy people. Another option is to do RLT at home, but ask a qualified medical expert for guidance before use.

"Red light devices are widely available and are very easy to manufacture," explains Arany. "They are also not terribly expensive." According to Arany, a knowledgeable practitioner is helpful for the success of red light therapy.

The more "exotic" you are in terms of health conditions, the more guidance you should seek. You might begin your RLT journey in a clinical setting such as a hospital or university.

Red light devices for skincare can be purchased and utilized at home. They are generally safe to use at home as long as you follow their instructions. They are typically not a powerful systemic treatment and they do not contain wavelengths of light that penetrating very deeply into the body. Even so, at these lower powers consumers report excellent results treating at home.

Applications of RLT

Patients may use red light therapy equipment, which includes handheld devices, LED panels, or even full-body beds containing LEDs in red, orange and invisible light wavelengths, depending on the condition they are treating. Some devices on the market use both near-infrared and red light.

Post & Pre-Therapy Effects of RLT

RLT is unlikely to be harmful, and it is known from a great deal of research over many decades to be non-invasive and safe. The majority of patients report no discomfort or pain during or after red light therapy sessions. You can press a portable gadget against the skin at a specific location on your body where treatment is required or where pain originates. You can experience pain relief and greater mobility from near-infrared bulbs in full-body beds or pods that employ red and near-infrared light, penetrating deeper into your muscles, tissue and at some wavelengths, even into your bones.

You may inquire about eye protection throughout treatment with the facilitating practitioner. All of the research done on RLT supports that it is not damaging to the eye. I personally do not use eye protection (nor do any of my colleagues) unless the brightness is too intense. With this said, it is your choice, dependant on your comfort level. In fact, the CEO of Theralight, Charles E. Vorwaller shared with me that users of their RLT beds have occasionally reported improved eyesight and less necessary vision correction with eyeglasses, but no formal studies done yet to date by Theralight have looked into this issue.

One of the most notable benefits of red light therapy is how relaxed patients feel following the treatment. Think of this time as yours, and immerse yourself in the calming effects.

Expect to require more than one treatment. Even if you are using RLT for anti-aging, it is like exercise; you will need to keep up if you expect the benefits to continue. Before starting therapy, talk to your healthcare provider to determine how many sessions you need and how frequently they should occur; this gives you a comprehensive understanding of the treatment's scope. In some cases, even a single treatment is effective.

A standard protocol for PBM treatment involves three sessions per week for a minimum of four weeks to observe significant effects. It is not surprising to find that a higher frequency of treatment leads to more noticeable results, especially as one begins RLT. I invited a physician to use my "Red Med Bed" while I was out of town. Mine has four wavelengths to target skin, the tissue beneath, organs, and bones. This MD went past my suggested use of one 20-minute session per day and did 2 sessions per day! He told me that it measurably transformed his energy level and digestive system and reduced his pain and inflammation; this was accomplished with 8 treatments in four days. He began as a "non-believer." He is now committed to these treatments but I was shocked that he initiated his treatment so aggressively. All I can say is that for him, it worked wonders, and now he enthusiastically does one maintenance session per day.

It is essential to keep in mind that the field of phototherapy is constantly advancing, and more research is required to find the most effective applications of various wavelengths, doses, and devices for treating particular diseases and ailments. If you have any questions before committing and investing in therapy, it is best to speak with a dermatologist, a pain specialist, or a physician that understands and focuses on cellular health rather than typical, traditional medicine. To determine whether or not red light therapy is right for you, your doctor can help weigh the benefits of the treatment against any potential adverse effects. I believe it is the most non-invasive and side effect free treatment for longevity and healing available.

Medical Use of RLT

The core effects of red and near-infrared light have been outlined in study after study, including the one that Dr. Michael Hamblin co-authored. These core effects include increased cell metabolism and energy production, which subsequent studies confirm as an essential component in assisting the body in the healing process.

In 2001, researchers sponsored by NASA improved on earlier NASA studies by exposing members of the United States Navy SEALs to red light. The outcome was wound healing at a much faster rate.

In 2002, the FDA (Food and Drug Administration) cleared a low-level laser therapy device, which opened the door for clinical uses of red light therapy in dermatology and the wellness business. It may be important to understand that it is possible to simply register a device with the FDA for low-risk usage. These FDA distinctions are not often understood. Clearing is far different than approval which is only granted with numerous clinical studies and data.

Researchers conducted a seminal study in 2008 and published it in the journal *Photomedicine and Laser Surgery* to fully understand the effects of RLT on the body. They discovered that red light exposure increased energy production in the mitochondria of cells, which beneficially impacts the cells' operation. Healthier cells make up a healthier body.

The benefits of red light treatment can be felt from head to toe, ranging from the restoration of hair and improved mood to the alleviation of chronic skin conditions, neuropathic pain, and the healing of muscles.

Even while the history of red light therapy is fascinating, more and more experts are concluding that natural healers using RLT are on the right track with their practices. Red and NIR light treatment panels currently on the market are among the most cutting-edge and accessible technology available, and this bodes well for the future.

There are devices or installations capable of simultaneously helping you undergo both Infra-red sauna treatment and red light therapy. Thanks to recent technological advances, LED light therapy has been taken to a higher level that may add additional detoxifying results. This natural treatment does not involve invasive procedures, and may be appropriate for many users.

We may consider LED therapy as the next evolutionary advancement in light therapy. Now you know that LED light therapy has the potential to be utilized for various purposes, ranging from specific applications to promoting overall wellness for the entire body. Healthier cells prevent the cascade of disease that inflammation brings. Restoring normal cellular function is life-altering.

Chapter 2: Difference Between RLT & NIR

Your cells are given energy by natural red light. LEDs inside a medical-grade red light therapy device, such as those manufactured by Joovv (as an example), deliver red and near-infrared wavelengths straight to your body. These natural photons of therapeutic light cause a chemical reaction in your cells' mitochondria, which stimulates energy production and regeneration of damaged tissue. In other words, RLT reduces oxidative stress in cells, and it enhances the generation of adenosine triphosphate (ATP), resulting in increased energy levels. Cellular respiration is responsible for converting food into usable energy as ATP. This chapter delves into the scientific aspects of light therapy and its crucial role in ATP generation. ATP is the cell's "energy currency".

Improved Cell Signaling

Specific wavelengths of light create a more favorable oxidative environment within your cells, leading to improved cellular respiration, cell functioning, and cell to cell signaling. Consequently, this leads to the activation of many intracellular metabolic pathways, an increase in protein synthesis, the activation of enzymes, and a faster progression through the cell cycle.

According to Jared Jagdeo, MD, founding director of the Center for Photomedicine at SUNY Downstate Health Sciences University in Brooklyn, New York, red light therapy (RLT) is a type of photomedicine. Photomedicine is "using light to treat skin and other health conditions." This hearkens back to Einstein, telling the world that the future of medicine lies in frequencies.

Having given you some background on RLT, there is more to understand about RLT's administration protocols. It would not be strange to think that the protocols for red light therapy may be in their infancy in 2023. We're still learning how to best use and deliver the light, but we know enough to keep it safe and to obtain great effects from it already.

RLT Products

Depending on the health condition or desired aesthetic result, patients can utilize red light therapy equipment containing LEDs in hand-held gadgets, masks, panels, or even full-body beds. The market offers a wide range of devices that utilize both red and near-infrared light.

LEDs or Lasers

Red light therapy is unlike other types of treatment because the treatment is not in the least uncomfortable. In fact, it's pretty much imperceptible- you don't feel a thing while it's being administered. Unlike lasers, RLT is NOT designed to injure or damage skin cells in order to get the desired outcome as the damaged tissue heals. By now, you may also understand that RLT is not just a treatment that works on the surface of the body. Depending on the wavelength and brightness of the light, it can penetrate beyond 50 millimeters below the skin's surface. The light can penetrate into the brain, improving mental clarity and offering many more benefits than we ever imagined. RLT derived from LEDs offers many benefits not shared by other types of treatment, such as cold or hot lasers. These treatments might result in discomfort, and they might also cause damage to the skin that subsequently needs to heal. Following an injury or dermal procedure that affects the outermost layer of skin, the body restores the damaged skin tissue. Lasers have significantly less treatment area when compared to products that use LEDs. This also explains why clinical laser treatments take longer than RLT treatments using LEDs. LED light disperses over a larger, less focused surface area, resulting in a shorter overall treatment times than lasers.

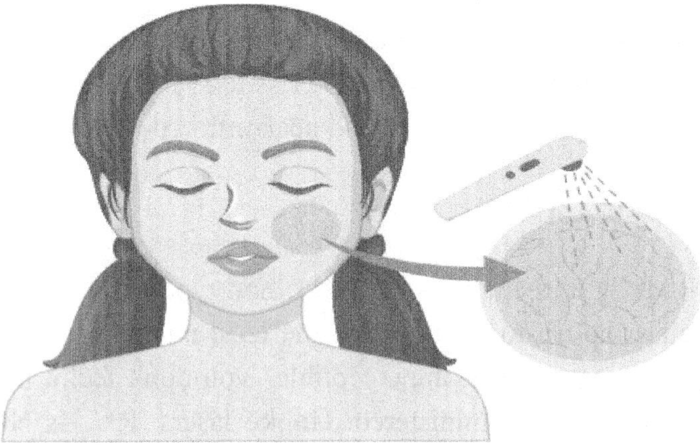

Red light treatment has the potential to provide a wide range of systemic advantages, including expedited muscle recovery, promotion of healthy skin, reduction of inflammation, enhancement of sleep quality, and alleviation of joint and muscle pain. These benefits, along with many others, are supported by a great deal of peer reviewed clinical research. RLT can be a fantastic healing agent after injuries and following medical or surgical procedures. Experienced clinicians suggest RLT after lasers to speed the healing process. Lasers are a more intense experience and not to be used frequently, as opposed to RLT, which can be used even daily.

How NIR light Works

Patients suffering from acute or chronic pain are candidates for several experimental treatments, and one of these is infrared light, with promising early results for many study subjects. IR light continues to be enthusiastically explored in the testing phase. The treatment involves directing specific wavelengths of light at the wounded areas of the body to promote faster, and often more complete, healing.

In contrast to UV light, which can harm both the tissues, cells, and even DNA, infrared light encourages the body's cells to repair or replenish themselves. Infrared light enhances the circulation of oxygen-rich blood throughout the body, expediting deep tissue healing and reducing pain.

Infrared light can penetrate deeper into the skin than other types of light, giving it broader reach in its capacity to alleviate pain. This non-invasive, natural, and painless modality delivers many advantages to one's health, without causing any damage to the skin, underlying tissues, or genetic material, all of which occur through exposure to ultraviolet light.

When exposed to infrared light from the sun, we feel warmth. The skin's surface naturally emits infrared heat daily. Infrared light offers significant health benefits, such as pain relief and inflammation reduction.

Treatment with Infrared light energy

The depth that infrared light can reach into the skin ranges from 2 to 7 cm. Because of this, it can affect muscles, nerves, and even bones. Numerous studies have demonstrated that the most effective method for treating inflammatory disorders is to administer infrared light with wavelengths ranging from 700 to 1,000 nanometers.

As early as 2,750 BC, people utilized electric eels to administer electric shocks to patients, marking the inception of electricity's use in medicine. The application of electricity and magnetism to individuals yielded moderate levels of success. In 1975, researchers created transcutaneous electrical stimulation (TENS) to treat chronic pain. More recently, infrared therapy has been developed to enhance wound healing, alleviate arthritis pain, and increase endorphin levels.

Through infrared treatment, individuals can get the benefits of the sun without being subjected to the sun's potentially dangerous ultraviolet radiation. Infrared therapy is not only beneficial but it also appears to be risk-free, as it does not have any adverse side effects that we can find.

Infrared light is therefore considered clinically harmless, and accepting its safety, many healthcare professionals utilize it to treat newborns. In stark contrast, it's well known that exposure to the white light from the sun, containing the whole spectrum of visible light, can lead to skin cancer. This is a result of exposure to the blue end of the visible

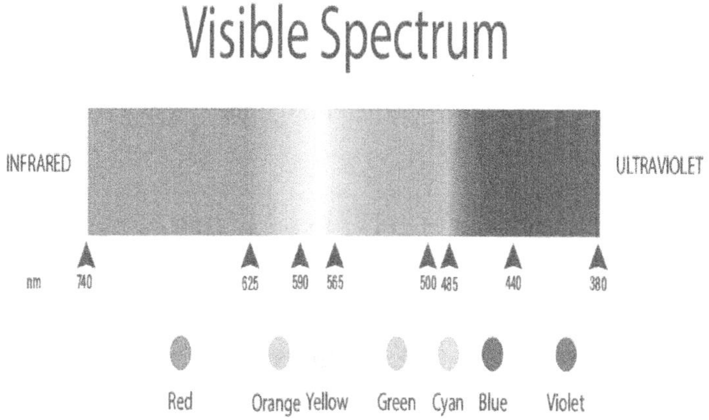

spectrum, leading off into violet light, ultraviolet light, and even X rays, as we move farther into shorter wavelengths of light energy. Again, on the other hand, basking in the red end of the visible spectrum of our sun's light, red, near infra-red, and true infrared light, is a health treatment. This can be done in the early morning and at sunset, or it can be simulated in a RLT device. By now this should be making sense!

Photoreceptors in cells can take in and process infrared light. After being absorbed, red light's energy sets off a chain of metabolic reactions within the cell, initiating and supporting many of the body's normal biologic functions.

It is possible that nitric oxide, a gas that is essential to the health of the body's arteries, is the element that is responsible for the effectiveness of infrared light therapy. Nitric oxide is a powerful cell signaling molecule that helps relax the smooth muscle in the walls of arteries. It fights free radicals to minimize oxidative stress, stops platelets from clumping together leading to blood clots, and it controls blood pressure by allowing the arteries to dilate. Nitric oxide improves blood circulation, which helps in the delivery of essential nutrients and oxygen tissues throughout the body.

With increased blood flow, oxygen and nutrients more easily reach the cells, enabling them to work more efficiently. This mechanism helps to explain how RLT promotes the regeneration and repair of wounded tissues, which results in a reduction in both pain and inflammation.

Medical professionals use infrared light therapy to treat a wide range of medical conditions such as arthritis, bursitis, blunt trauma, muscle strain, carpal tunnel syndrome, neck pain, back pain, diabetic neuropathy, rheumatoid arthritis, temporomandibular joint pain (TMJ), tendonitis, chronic wounds, sciatica, and surgical incisions. People with back pain may benefit greatly from infrared light therapy, and they may use it as an alternative to potentially addictive narcotic pain medications.

The following are some well accepted conclusions regarding infrared therapy.

Infrared treatment is a non-invasive and highly successful method for treating many illnesses, including any of them that result in pain. RLT appears to be safe and effective (a highly desirable combination), and it accomplishes this without drugs and their inevitable side effects. It is also known to help wounded tissue heal faster, as previously stated, most likely through modulation of nitric oxide.

RLT for injuries offers several benefits, mostly derived through the reduction of inflammation. Restoration of normal function to an injured area of the body can be attributed to this anti-inflammatory effect. Through this mechanism, RLT can effectively treat many illnesses and injuries.

Benefits of NIR Therapy

The wavelength of light used in near-infrared (NIR) light treatment falls between 800 to 1100 nm, which places it just outside the visible light spectrum. RLT is categorized into these two forms/colors of light, red and near infra-red.

I recommended full-body RLT to a physician that manages his chronic pain with his mind, avoiding pharmaceuticals. The "Med Bed" that we own, which contains 4 wavelengths of red and NIR light, has alleviated most of his chronic pain that he's had since childhood. Prior to this RLT, he used to refer to chronic pain as 'background noise'. It was just a reality that he chose to ignore, unless it became so severe that the noise drowned out everything else. More recently, with RLT, the background noise appears to be much softer.

In this chapter, we explore the positive effects of NIR therapy and compare them to those of other red light therapy. We offer the three main advantages of utilizing near-infrared light.

Advantages for Skincare

Near infra-red light promotes cellular activity, enabling the skin to regenerate and mend, improving its appearance, its feel, and its texture.

The following section elaborates further on this topic: NIR light aids in skin healing following an injury. Furthermore, it possesses anti-aging properties that benefit the skin. The longer wavelength of NIR light increases the production of collagen and elastin in the skin, both of which play a crucial role in maintaining its youthful appearance, which we all want!

CEO and President of Clearskin Institute in Phoenix, Arizona, Larry Helwig, specializes in all phases of non-surgical aesthetics. He has developed some of the best aesthetic practices for treating with lasers and RLT in the country. Helwig told me, "The one with the most collagen wins!" I know he uses this premise to support the use of RLT and also has a large RLT pod available to his clientele.

Aging concerns that may bother nearly everyone over the age of 40 include wrinkles, sagging, decreased elasticity, roughness, and poor texture of the skin. Before considering surgery, it is worth trying Red Light Therapy. RLT is also frequently recommended in surgical recovery to speed the healing process.

Anti-Inflammatory Process

Continuous inflammation is one of the issues that might develop due to excessive oxidative stress. Even though some inflammation serves a therapeutic purpose, such as in the immune system's defense against infection, excessive inflammation leads to many health issues including cancer and cardio-vascular disease, which are the number one and number two killers in humans. Excess inflammation is known to be the root cause of most diseases. NIR therapy provides cellular energy and expands blood vessels, which counteracts the generation of excess inflammation.

Healing Wounds

NIR therapy speeds wound healing in various ways, including those not limited to the skin. Collagen synthesis speeds up the healing process and reduces the appearance of scars with RLT. RLT's benefits extend deeper than the skin's surface.

The natural healing process that your body goes through can mend itself after suffering from acute injuries, painful muscles, joint and muscle discomfort, minor muscle damage, or repetitive trauma.

RLT can be applied locally to the affected area or utilized as a part of overall body treatment by assisting the body's innate capacity for repair and restoration.

NIR light therapy promotes healing in multiple ways, including reducing inflammation and improving circulation. RLT has been shown to be more effective than ice therapy, which inhibits the early, 'good' inflammation that is required for early wound healing. Ice may therefore slow the overall healing process, in contrast to RLT, which is known to speed it up!

Full-Body Photobiomodulation

Photobiomodulation therapy is another term that utilizes therapeutic light encouraging beneficial life-changing processes, most easily implemented in a "Med Bed" such as the one that I use daily, which is large; it looks like a commercial tanning bed. As I've explained, it produces four wavelengths of red to infrared light. I simultaneously treat skin, underlying tissue and muscle, bones, and organs.

It is possible to apply near-infrared light therapy to a smaller, more limited region, such as the face or the site of an injury. With exception to pregnant mothers or in utero fetuses, it is my strong belief that RLT is very advantageous and most effective when applied to the entire body; it becomes a systemic treatment rather than a local one. With this treatment, the whole body benefits.

Individualized Methods

Photo-therapy provides the flexibility to adapt to each patient's specific objectives and requirements. Various treatment techniques are available for light therapy to deliver the maximum advantage. A provider of light treatment can select the light wavelength, such as near-infrared light, but they can also select continuous- or pulsed- light.

Wave treatments may offer a lower power, ongoing session, or pulsed wave treatments that produce rapid bursts of more potent energy. Subjects suffering from chronic headaches and other similar neurologic issues prefer wave treatments that do not flicker. A clinician can provide therapy for a predetermined amount of time throughout each session, as well as make suggestions on the treatment's frequency and duration to accommodate your care plan. That plan becomes personalized, based on whether your objective is to enhance your health, improve the appearance of your skin, or recover from an injury.

Comparison of NIR to RLT

Red light therapy and near-infrared light therapy belong to a completely different portion of the light spectrum. The two are frequently considered very similar; however, there is a significant difference between them. On the electromagnetic scale, red light, which ranges in wavelength from 630 to 700 nanometers, belongs to the visible portion of the light spectrum and is the type of light used to treat the skin's surface. Near-infrared wavelengths, ranging between 700 and 1200 nanometers, exist in the portion of the electromagnetic spectrum that is not visible to humans. What does this imply? The longer the wavelength, the deeper the energy may penetrate to transfer energy to the cells, accelerating healing and decreasing pain. There are many different types of cells and tissues, each with its unique way of absorbing light at a particular wavelength; this indicates that different types of tissues absorb different wavelengths of light. Light with a wavelength of red benefits the skin, although the light of other colors may penetrate the skin more deeply while as we all know, other wavelengths of light actually damage the skin. Other LED colors are used in many ways for skin treatment but red and near-infra-red light is the focus of this book.

LED technology is the best option for NIR applications because you can adjust the surface temperature and keep the subject from feeling hot. LEDs scatter their light over a broader surface area than halogen bulbs or lasers. The mode in which light energy is delivered (optical power output – OPD) is another significant distinction between LEDs, halogen bulbs, and lasers. As we keep stressing for effect, near-infrared energy, ranging between 700 and 1200 nanometers, exists in the portion of the electromagnetic spectrum that is not visible to us. Interestingly, because of this, LEDs that deliver NIR light don't 'look' like they're on. I initially thought that half of the LEDs in my Med-Bed didn't work.

Research conducted by NASA has shown that the electromagnetic frequency band known as NIR can travel very deep into the body and potentially have a curative effect on cells. Some receptors are sensitive to near-infrared wavelengths within each cell's mitochondria. An increase in

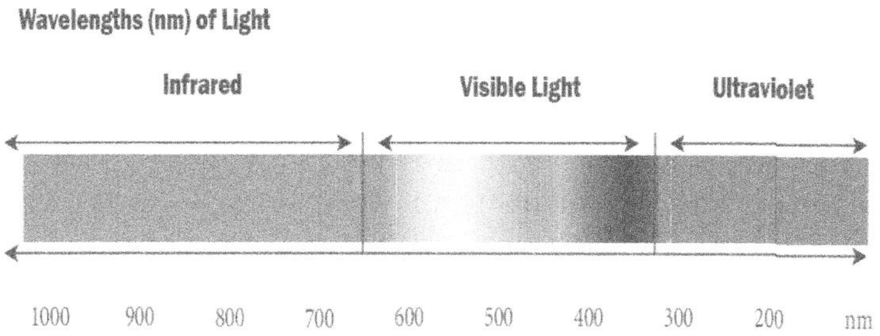

cellular metabolism, protein synthesis (including the production of collagen), and anti-oxidant activity (which means the cells detoxify) are all prompted by NIR. It lessens inflammation and pain while simultaneously stimulating the growth and regeneration of cells.

Light therapy affects mood, circadian rhythm, and other bodily functions, whereas near-infrared treatment acts as a pain reliever and cell rejuvenator. These are two VERY distinct, but HIGHLY SYNERGISTIC forms of energy!!

Chapter 3: Benefits of RLT for Humans

Medical specialists tend to consider red light therapy as complementary to mainstream treatments; it is typically expected to be used alongside traditional and approved modalities. For instance, if you have fine lines and wrinkles, you might benefit from red light therapy along with dermatologist-prescribed topicals, retinoids, or in-office laser treatments. If you sustain an injury while playing sports, your physical therapist or chiropractor may suggest red light therapy. The following data contains some potential health benefits that red light treatment may offer your regular healthcare practice in general.

Skin, Hair, Acne & Wrinkles

One of the most common applications of red light therapy is its use in treating skin diseases. RLT is also utilized for beautification of normal or aging skin. The growing accessibility is driving the RLT market through newly achieved popularity and perceived results. Below is a list of conditions that red light can effectively treat.

Wrinkles and skin lines: Researchers assert that red light therapy has the potential to treat and prevent wrinkles and lines. Red light is shown to activate collagen, which in turn may help smooth out wrinkles and creases. Note that you may have better luck with lines that are modest and minimal as opposed to those that are already profoundly carved in, such as nasal labial folds. You will most likely require additional treatments in conjunction with red light depending on the severity of your condition.

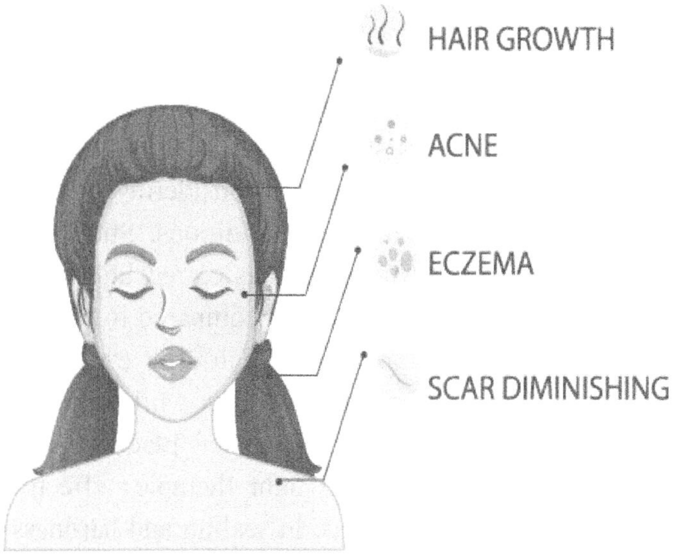

Acne breakouts persist as those who are prone to it age. Many people struggle with both acne and the signs of aging. You may be able to treat both conditions simultaneously with measurable results. A small controlled clinical trial published in January 2022 in the journals *Photodermatology, Photoimmunology,* and *Photomedicine* demonstrated that red light therapy reduced the number of acne lesions by 36% in patients with mild to moderate acne. The mechanism to explain how this works is that red light therapy helps to reduce inflammation and it may assist in killing bacteria, two established factors contributing to the development of acne.

Redness: For some, it goes against standard thinking that red light would effectively reduce skin redness; one of the critical purposes of red light is to reduce inflammation. Having less inflammation in the skin might help to reduce erythema, or skin redness. The NCCIH (National Center for Complementary and Integrative Health) states that there is insufficient evidence to establish the usefulness of red light in treating skin disorders such as psoriasis. Unfortunately, there is a lack of sufficient studies considering the use of red light as a treatment for such conditions. Studies have been conducted to identify the effects of red light therapy (RLT) on individuals with psoriasis compared to blue light therapy. The participants received high-dose treatments 3 times per week for 4 consecutive weeks while applying a 10 percent salicylic acid solution to their plaques. Results showed that the red and blue light therapies effectively treated psoriasis. The difference in scaling and hardness of the plaques between the two treatment arms was insignificant. Blue light, however, did work better when treating erythema alone. It is crucial to remember that medical personnel administered these treatments in high doses. Therapy at home, a salon, or a wellness center, may not yield such striking outcomes, as the power/doses delivered are typically smaller.

Hair growth using red light continues to be another common therapy for hair loss. Red light helps decrease inflammation and promotes more blood flow to the scalp and hair, which allows follicles to get more oxygen and nutrients. Blue light helps decrease inflammation and promotes blood flow to the hair and scalp in a similar manner. In July 2020, *Skin Appendage Disorders* published a literature review of 10 controlled studies on low-level laser therapy (LLLT) using red and near-infrared light. This treatment demonstrated increased hair density and thickness compared to other invasive surgeries and was safe, with minor side effects limited to scalp itching.

The potential for red light to alleviate pain associated with various chronic diseases is the subject of ongoing research. Praveen Arany, Ph.D., says, "Red light does help with pain." Red light therapies can reduce inflammation and pain if you use the proper protocol and he demonstrated that red light clearly possesses anti-inflammatory and anti-pain properties. How so? A protein on the neuron's surface inhibits the cell's ability to conduct or sense pain when it absorbs light. From a complementary perspective, red light therapy is beneficial for treating pain, as it is non-addictive and has relatively no side effects. If it can reduce, or better yet, eliminate the need for pain medications, then it has tremendous value as a compliment to traditional approaches.

Athletic Performance

Exposure to red light may stimulate mitochondria, the "energy powerhouses" of cells, triggering an enzyme that drives production of ATP, referred to as "energy currency." In the end, this can be beneficial for muscle growth and repair. According to research published in *AIMS Biophysics* in 2017, photobiomodulation treatment (PBM) using red or near-infrared light before exercise may boost muscular function, heal muscle injury, and reduce post-workout discomfort and soreness.

The Healing Process

Red light can effectively treat various types of wounds, including those on the skin and mouth. In such situations, the medical staff would treat the region of the wound with red light until the healing is complete. A preliminary study conducted on animals and published in July 2021 in the journal *Photobiomodulation, Photomedicine, and Laser Surgery* suggests that RLT may also be helpful for burns. Another study published in May 2022 in the journal *BMC Oral Health* indicates that PBM can also be helpful in healing wounds after oral surgery. PBM also improves cell function, hastens tissue regeneration, reduces inflammation and pain, and stimulates the release of growth factors, among other benefits for quicker healing.

Cancer Treatment & RLT

Oral mucositis is a potential side effect that can occur as a result of chemotherapy or radiation therapy. This condition can cause pain, ulcers, infections, and bleeding inside the mouth. According to a comprehensive study that appeared in the August 2022 issue of *Frontiers in Oncology*, PBM can help to prevent and treat this complication. According to a review published in June 2019 in the journal *Oral Oncology*, photobiomodulation

(PBM) has been used successfully on skin damage caused by radiation treatments and lymphedema following mastectomy. The light therapy did not create any additional adverse effects during these treatments. PBM is a potential complimentary cancer treatment because it may either increase the body's immune response or enhance the effectiveness of existing cancer treatments in helping to kill cancer cells.

In 2023, Praveen Arany explained to me in an interview that PBM supports cancer care. There is no evidence that PBM will increase tumor growth or stimulate cancer cells. It is non-ionizing radiation. It is likely that PBM helps diseased cells to "commit suicide." This genetically controlled programmed cell death is termed Apoptosis. It is actually a natural part of the aging process. Apoptosis is your friend in the case of cancer cells, but it is your enemy in the face of brain cells as we age, or the Leydig cells in the testicles that produce testosterone, as two examples. It easily becomes clear that Apoptosis can be good or it can be bad. The ability to modulate it is therefore intriguing! RLT does exactly that.

RLT is Non-Invasive

Doctors commonly use cortisone injections to treat joint discomfort caused by arthritis or tendonitis. In this treatment, they inject a corticosteroid into the affected joint. Without this injection, it is common for the patient to experience worsening pain and inflammation within the first forty-eight hours following an operation. At the same time, red light therapy does not involve any discomfort. Your body naturally absorbs the light, correctly dosed and calibrated by a health specialist, to your needs.

Photobiomodulation therapy is not only a treatment that does not cause any discomfort, but it is also relaxing. Beds that use red light therapy, such as TheraLight 360 and FIT, are becoming increasingly popular. The bed is designed with a cooling capability to dissipate the heat, which is minimal anyway with the light being generated by LED's. This ensures that the treatments remain comfortable. Red light therapy treatments are between three and twenty minutes long, providing the user with some much-needed downtime as it provides a healing light for your body and mind. A PBM treatment can be a fantastic opportunity to disengage for a few minutes and focus solely on yourself and your health.

No Adverse Effect

Over-the-counter pain drugs like ibuprofen, acetaminophen, and naproxen are standard therapeutic options for managing pain and to some degree, inflammation. While these medications are available without a doctor's prescription, they all have significant undesirable side effects. If taken consistently for several weeks or months, ibuprofen can cause stomach pain, nausea, and kidney failure. Acetaminophen (Tylenol) can cause damage to the liver if taken for an extended period or in high doses.

Cortisone injections can cause further degradation of joint cartilage, ligaments, and even bone. Due to these side effects, healthcare providers sometimes (and truly always should) restrict the amount of pain medication that they recommend or prescribe. One of the most significant advantages of red light therapy is that it does not produce any long-term or potentially dangerous side effects. Most people are in and out of the office in less than half an hour, and then they can continue their day as usual. Some patients experience lightheadedness upon rising, and healthcare providers and patients should simply be aware of this. People who are light-sensitive or take medications that make them more light-sensitive are not encouraged to use RLT.

Combining RLT with Other Treatments

Another advantage of PBM treatment is that healthcare providers can use it with diet, exercise, and other therapies, such as physical and occupational therapy. Hyperbaric oxygen therapy and stem cell therapy are well complemented by RLT. Combining red light therapy with other treatments can yield more successful results than using either red light therapy or the primary treatment alone.

Individual Treatments

Exercise: The benefits of RLT extend beyond reducing inflammation and alleviating pain. It can be helpful in many situations, even if you aren't currently dealing with pain. A full-body red light treatment before a workout improves circulation and helps warm the body for vigorous exercise, reducing the risk of injury. After a strenuous workout or competition, red light treatment can help minimize the effects of DOMS (delayed onset muscular soreness) by healing micro-tears in muscle fibers. Treating to energize your cells before performance or after a workout to recover is possible with red light therapy.

Skincare: Red light treatment naturally increases collagen production, which can assist in the healing of wounds and prevent the formation of scar tissue. Red light therapy treats various skin conditions, including acne, wrinkles, and fine lines; this is because red light therapy stimulates the creation of collagen. An increase in collagen production enhances suppleness of the skin overall. It can help to reduce the appearance of acne scarring and redness by addressing inflammation. Many of my friends and colleagues choose to use their RLT masks before bed. After cleansing the skin, red light therapy in the evening can help signal the body to release melatonin, improving mood and sleep quality.

Sleep: The blue light emitted from computer screens and the white fluorescent lights found in many workplaces can disrupt our circadian rhythms, making sleeping more difficult. Red light therapy can assist in correcting this disruption, thereby improving sleep patterns.

Advantages of RLT for the Body

Healthcare providers administer light to the entire body during a full-body red light session; this helps reduce inflammation and addresses underlying conditions that may not be immediately apparent, such as oxidative stress. The imbalance between antioxidants and free radicals results in oxidative stress, making it easier for free radicals to damage cells. Healthy cells are susceptible to being affected by external elements such as pollution. The development of aging symptoms, such as wrinkles, has been linked to oxidative stress. In addition to more severe problems such as diabetes, cancer, and inflammatory illnesses, a red light treatment administered to the entire body can help reverse the damage caused by free radicals and restore a healthy balance between them and antioxidants. Even if you're not sick, red light treatment paired with a nutritious diet and a consistent workout routine can benefit a lifestyle that prioritizes health.

Psychological Advantages of RLT

You won't be able to enjoy life to its fullest if you're struggling with depression, mood disorders, and anxiety. Long, dark winter months cause depression and limit clarity of the mind. You can get through these challenges with the help of the appropriate treatments. Light therapy is one of the most effective and safest methods for treating different types of depression and illnesses related to fatigue, anxiety, and seasonal affective disorder (SAD). Around five percent of the population in the United States suffers from SAD.

Those living in parts of the world that do not receive a significant amount of natural light during the winter months are at risk of developing it. "SAD lamps" emit a bright, artificial light that simulates natural sunlight. These lights can illuminate a dark space and create the illusion of natural light. However, they still contain a significant amount of blue light, which can disrupt your circadian rhythm, cause fatigue, and even damage delicate structures in your eyes. A safer and likely more effective approach is RLT.

Benefits of RLT for Brain Health

Applying light to one's head through a full body pod, a helmet, or some other device, offers potential benefits of red light therapy for the brain. There is striking evidence that shows photobiomodulation treatments improve neurocognition. According to an article published in the *Journal of Neuroscience Research* in April 2018, PBM may reduce inflammation and improve blood flow and oxygen delivery to the brain. This may help to form new neurons and synapses (the connections between neurons that allow them to communicate with one another); this may be helpful for people who have suffered traumatic brain injuries or strokes. With more ongoing studies and targeted treatments, we are witnessing more advances in the neurologic application of RLT.

Treating Depression with RLT

Mental illnesses such as depression, anxiety, and bipolar disorder negatively impact today's society significantly. The use of red light therapy shows great promise in treating mental health conditions, as previously mentioned in conjunction with SAD. Patients diagnosed with major depressive disorder exhibited a significant response to the antidepressant effects of RLT. Light therapy offers a "promising treatment" for suicidal ideation, depressive disorder, anxiety, and traumatic brain injury.

Even though light is everywhere, most of us don't give it much thought on a daily basis. The extent to which light satisfies our fundamental requirements and supports our bodily functions is something that we take for granted. More than enough evidence is now available to suggest that exposure to natural light is essential to our well-being and that a deficiency in this aspect of our environment can significantly affect our health. With a deficit of adequate natural light, or if one desires the positive, healing effect while limiting the damaging effects from natural light, red light therapy is a great way to supplement the void.

Even if it is already dark outside when you arrive home from work, you may still create the health enhancing effects of light exposure by using red light therapy equipment. You may gain the benefit of a whole day's natural light, while eliminating the potentially harmful effects from the other end of the electromagnetic spectrum, in as little as ten to fifteen minutes with an RLT device.

The same goes for an occasional rainy day, or a very rainy climate, where adequate light exposure is lacking. The simplicity and low risk involved in red light therapy supplementation in these settings has led to the medical community more widely accepting it as a supplement and even as a treatment for seasonal depression. Forward-thinking doctors who share this view already use natural light therapy for depression. Anyone using red light therapy should monitor or journal how their feelings and moods are affected, and it's wise to discuss this or related questions with a physician or a licensed health professional.

Chapter 4: RLT for Pets

Red light therapy is a straightforward and non-invasive treatment for pets and horses as well. RLT can treat many illnesses, ranging from acute injuries to chronic conditions such as arthritis. This treatment is becoming increasingly popular in the veterinary community. This chapter answers the following questions:

- What positive effects does RLT have on the health of animals?
- How do you administer RLT to a pet in your own home?
- Is the treatment with red light safe for pets?
- What exactly is meant by the term "red light therapy," and how is it applied to animals?

Red light therapy is the technique of beaming therapeutic red and near-infrared (NIR) penetrating light onto animals to improve their overall health and well-being, exactly the same as in its application to humans. This type of light can help treat a wide variety of conditions, as it does for humans. RLT is a safer alternative to medications for pets. Photobiomodulation (PBM), low-power laser therapy (LPLT), and low-level laser treatment (LLLT), are synonyms for red light therapy.

Over the past decade, veterinarians have increasingly turned to red light therapy (RLT) as a treatment option. In animal rehabilitation settings, practitioners commonly utilize red light therapy to treat pain and inflammation, and for the management of chronic wounds. As with humans, RLT is commonly used by veterinarians for the treatment of arthritis, the control of chronic pain, and the mending of injuries.

Several veterinarians still administer red light therapy using low-level lasers. Due to advancements in LED technology, red light treatment crates such as Glowbie are now on the market and may be used by pet owners on their animals at home. The Glowbie crate illuminates using light-emitting diode or LED lights that emit red light in the range of 660 nm and near-infrared light in the range of 850 nm. The vast majority of animals can relax and enjoy Glowbie sessions. With as little as a few sessions per week, you may notice changes in your pet's health including increased energy and mobility and reduced discomfort and inflammation.

Early Animal Trials of RLT

In the 1960s, therapeutic trials of red light treatment began with animals as the test subjects. Dr. Endre Mester was the first to demonstrate these therapies, including light therapy. In 1967, Dr. Mester found that mice given wavelengths of red light experienced significantly increased rates of new hair growth compared to those not given the treatment. Horse trainers were among the first animal owners to use red light treatment techniques. These techniques involve the utilization of red and NIR light to assist horses in recovering from tendon and ligament injuries.

Since the 1990s, veterinarians have used a variety of forms of red light therapy. Still, it has become substantially more widespread in the last ten years as approximately twenty percent of clinics employ some form of photobiomodulation (PBM) treatment. Medical organizations are publishing guidelines for effective red light therapy treatments for dogs and cats to standardize the practice of red light therapy. In modern veterinary medicine, red light therapy is one of the treatment techniques experiencing the most rapid expansion.

Treating Pets with RLT

Red light therapy helps animals regenerate tissues and manufacture energy more efficiently at the cellular level. This is the most basic explanation for how this treatment can benefit dogs. To generate power and keep their bodies functioning, animals of every size require a steady supply of food, water, oxygen, and light; all animals accomplish this through cellular respiration, which creates ATP, or adenosine triphosphate, which, as explained earlier, is 'energy currency'.

Mitochondria in animal cells can absorb specific wavelengths of red and near-infrared light. The use of red light therapy can result in an increase in the number of mitochondria in mammalian cells as well as an improvement in their function. The photons of red light stimulate electrons in the mitochondria, which helps to eliminate toxic nitric oxide (NO). NO is known to slow down the process of cellular respiration. As with humans, RLT therefore assists an animal's cells to produce more ATP, which in turn helps power the body and its healing processes.

Treatments with red light can enhance blood flow and modulate an animal's inflammatory response and immune system. Because it encourages an animal's body to produce more of the essential components of the healing process, red light is an effective treatment for wounds and injuries sustained by pets. The production of growth factors within an animal's body, which is essential to the production of new skin cells, fibroblasts, and collagen, is stimulated by wavelengths of red and NIR light. Red light treatments can enhance the activity of osteoblasts, essential bone cells required for recovery after fractures and other types of bone injuries.

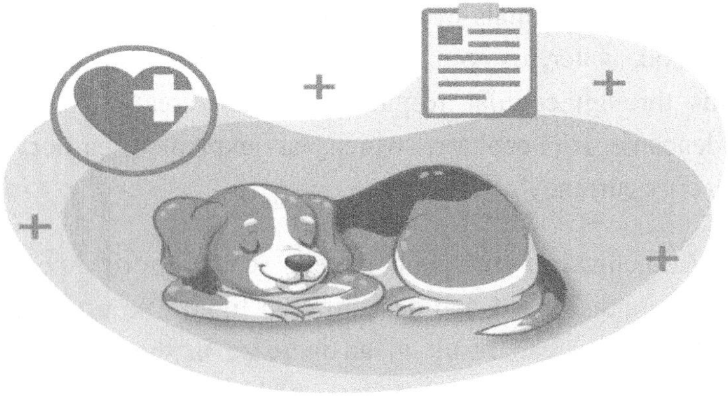

Health Benefits for Pets Using RLT

In animal rehabilitation facilities, red light therapy is frequently used to expedite the healing process and aid animals in recovery from injuries and traumatic experiences. A prospective study conducted in 2012 assessed the medical records of 36 dogs that had undergone spine surgery for the treatment of intervertebral disk herniation. This study was one of the earliest controlled trials conducted on companion pets. While one group of dogs was given red light therapy for 5 days following surgery, the control group did not receive any post-operative light treatment. The researchers came to the conclusion that the dogs that were given red light therapy after surgery were able to walk again after the procedure more quickly and with less discomfort than the dogs that did not receive RLT.

Veterinarians and pet owners utilize red light treatment to alleviate pain and inflammation, speed the healing process following injuries, and treat chronic illnesses like arthritis. The following section provides an analysis of the positive effects that red light treatment can have on the health of animals.

Recently my dog, Jewell, had puppies by C-section, and her large belly scar healed quickly and invisibly within 2 months with a few short (5-10 minute) RLT treatments each week. I witnessed no discomfort and she now begs to get into my RLT pod whenever I open it.

Avoiding Pain Medication for Animals

Veterinarians employ red light therapy as a non-pharmaceutical method for pain control. Red light therapy and NIR light can exert an analgesic impact, reducing pain in one study done on injured cats. The findings from that study were just as we've already discussed for humans. The evidence shows that our extensive experience with humans can confidently be extrapolated to other animals, as common sense would dictate.

Treating Canine Skin Issues

Silky, short-coated breeds such as English Bulldogs, Dachshunds, Great Danes, and Boxers, exhibit a high incidence of recurring skin issues and inflammation around the paws. A recent study was conducted on dogs afflicted with podo-dermatitis (inflammation in the skin of the paw) to determine the effectiveness of red light therapy for healing skin sores. Between the fourth and twentieth day following the onset of a lesion, they observed that dogs treated with red light therapy displayed significantly more signs of healing than untreated dogs. More than half of the dogs who underwent red light treatment for podo-dermatitis did not encounter any recurrence of lesions, and there were no reports of severe side effects.

Osteoarthritis & Arthritis

Due to its high success rate, veterinarians widely use red light therapy to treat osteoarthritis and joint discomfort in older pets. A recent survey conducted in the United States among veterinarians showed that 43% of respondents used red light therapy to treat canine patients with arthritis. The use of red light therapy is expected to grow as more pet owners become aware of RLT's benefits for older dogs and cats with joint problems. Increasing numbers of veterinarians recognize the advantages of RLT treatment.

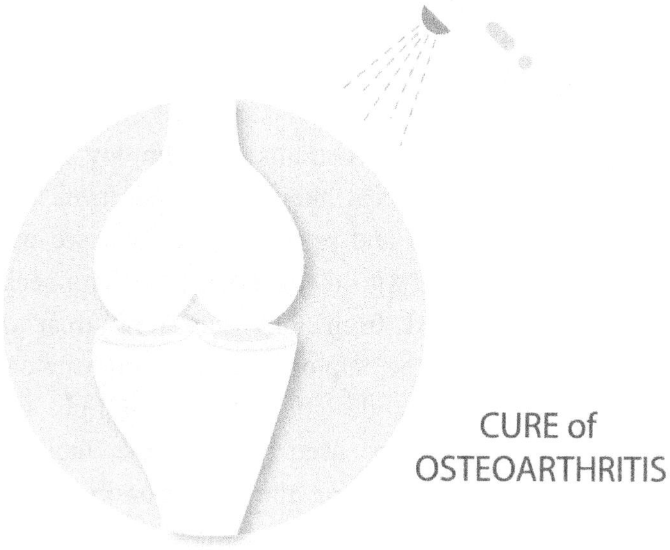

Effects of Proactive RLT for Cats & Dogs

Red light therapy is being used on animals by many veterinarians and pet owners as a preventative measure to improve the animals' overall health and well-being. There is a possibility that animals that routinely undergo red light therapy would experience improved skin and coat quality, enhanced bone and joint health, higher quality of sleep, more energy to play and enhanced cognitive function.

RLT as Veterinary Medicine

The field of veterinary medicine has recognized red light therapy as a method for improving the health of companion animals. Veterinary health experts are using low-level lasers and red light LED technology as treatments for acute injuries, therapies for chronic illnesses, and preventative health and wellness aids.

Using RLT for Pets at Home

Most of the time, veterinarians who employ red light treatment on animals treat them with low-level lasers. These are cumbersome and pricey devices that are out of reach for most people who own pets. Pet owners seeking the benefits described from RLT can now treat their animals at home with the help of a lower cost device called the Glowbie crate. The design of these red light crates enables them to easily be used in the home, facilitating continuous pet treatment for the best possible results. Treating a pet three to four times per week is recommended for optimal results. Consistency is one of the most important factors when it comes to the efficacy of red light treatment for an animal, just as it is for humans.

RLT Safety Regarding Pets

Red light therapy poses little to no danger to animals as a treatment, again, consistent with the results for humans, as we would expect. LED systems, such as the ones used in Glowbie kennels, are exceptionally safe and have a high level of acceptance and enthusiasm among customers. Red light therapy should not be used on some animals with sensitivities, just as it should be avoided in certain human cases, because it can cause specific light and photosensitivity issues. It is strongly discouraged to administer RLT to animals that are prone to seizures. Before treating animals with active malignancy, examining the treatment options with a reputable veterinarian is recommended. After consulting with several CEO's and Founders of RLT device companies, I am told consistently that eye protection is not needed for pets. In fact, the vast majority of dogs cannot see red light at all, as their visible spectrum is thought to be narrow compared to that of humans.

Laser Light Therapy for Horses

In human and veterinary medicine, photobiomodulation with lasers has established itself as one of the most effective treatment modalities. A laser emits light with a specific focal point, radiating at a specific wavelength and frequency, to achieve optimal tissue penetration and deliver the most beneficial biological effect.

Because the laser stimulates the cell's metabolism, the amount of ATP (adenosine triphosphate), the primary energy source for all cell functions, increases. As a result of this stimulation, the body experiences increased tissue repair and cellular regeneration, leading to enhanced circulation, accelerated healing, and reduced pain levels.

Types of Lasers Used on Horses

We categorize lasers into groups based on their potential to cause eye damage rather than their effect on other tissue types.

- Class 1 lasers cannot cause any harm to the eye.
- Class 2 lasers have the potential to cause eye injury, but only if the exposure is prolonged and direct.
- Class 3 lasers provide an energy output ranging from one to five hundred milliwatts (mW), and they are capable of causing eye injury with prolonged exposure.
- Class 4 lasers have a higher energy output, emitting at 500 mW or higher. If mishandled, these lasers have the potential to cause rapid and significant damage to the eye, as well as other tissues.

Class 1 and 3 lasers, also known as low-level or cold lasers, and Class 4 lasers, also known as high-power or regenerative lasers, are frequently used on horses.

Cold laser therapy has proven beneficial in accelerating wound healing. They are widely used for treating injuries to tendons and ligaments in race horses. Incorrect use of a regenerative laser can cause damage since it is more powerful and emits light at a longer wavelength than other lasers. Because of this, only veterinarians are allowed to use Class 4 lasers, which require special precautions to prevent burns to the skin and eyes.

Wavelength & Frequency of the Laser

The tissue response is affected by the laser's wavelength and the frequency of the light pulses. For instance, to treat tissues like a tendon injury, a wavelength of 900 nanometers (nm) penetrates the epidermis most effectively because of its longer waves. When it comes to healing more superficial wounds, a wavelength of 470 nanometers is the one that has the least amount of penetration deep to the skin.

Compared to a frequency of 250 MHz, a laser frequency of 2000 MHz is more effective for relieving pain, but it also results in slower tissue healing. Your veterinarian uses these considerations to devise a laser therapy program tailored to the particular injury sustained by an animal, in our current conversation, a horse.

- Advantages of Cold Laser Therapy for Horses
- Reduces swelling and inflammation
- Increases blood flow and lymphatic flow
- Promotes faster wound healing
- Reduces the amount of time needed for tissue regeneration
- Assists in the removal of waste from cells
- Methods for Utilizing Cold Lasers on Horses
- The type of injury and the precise laser determine the frequency and number of sessions.

Always gaze at a laser from a safe distance while wearing protective eye-wear; no matter what, don't look directly into a laser.

The length of the horse's coat and the color of its skin will both affect the laser's ability to penetrate into the animal.

Some examples of Laser Therapy in the barn include the following:

- Complementary treatment for injuries to the tendons or ligaments, such as tearing, tendinitis, or desmitis (a very common inflammation of the long suspensory ligaments in horse's legs)
- Lasers promote wound healing by stimulating growth factors and collagen formation, and they also help prevent infection at the wound's surface.

Benefits of RLT for Horses

The therapeutic application of visible and invisible light is called light therapy (phototherapy). The full spectrum encompasses potentially hazardous wavelengths, including gamma rays and X-rays, alongside wavelengths visible to the human eye, and radio waves.

Although this particular form of light therapy can only penetrate the skin by about 1/8 of an inch (or 5 mm), the heat generated by the light can reach much deeper when used to treat tissues located close to the skin's surface. Red light is both visible and effective. In contrast, infrared light is not visible to the human eye and has a slightly longer wavelength. Because of this, infrared light penetrates deeper into the body than visible red light, which in turn can penetrate deeper than, for example, blue light, with an even shorter wavelength. LEDs, or light-emitting diodes, are the devices of choice for producing this therapy light.

RLT & Other Light Therapies

When it comes to laser and light therapy, enough information on the topic exists to fill an entire library of books. Instrument and modality names are often interchanged in the literature, leading to a great deal of confusion. Examples I've run across in researching the subject include:

- Laser light therapy with a low-power setting
- Laser treatment with low power
- LED lighting that doesn't become hot.
- Laser with an infrared wavelength
- Phototherapy using a laser
- Therapy with a gentle laser
- Laser treatment, therapeutic

Etc...

Both laser beams and LEDs can stimulate cells within the body. A laser emits a coherent light beam. The light beam of this type consists of waves with identical frequencies and exhibits a high concentration level. This one-of-a-kind coherent light emits a concentrated beam that travels straight and is collimated to reach deeper tissues. Because the red and infrared light emitted by LEDs is non-coherent, it is most effective for treating more superficial tissues.

Red light therapy uses wavelengths that are visible to the human eye, whereas the human eye cannot perceive the light emitted from cold lasers. Several companies have created devices that emit hybrids of laser and non-coherent light to increase the ease and accuracy of laser aiming.

Conclusion

Red light therapy for treating pets is proven effective and safe, and it is being used by veterinarians more and more and investigated by researchers. The use of red light therapy can assist animals in experiencing less pain and inflammation, in addition to accelerating recovery from injuries and procedures. It is also an efficient treatment for persistent conditions such as arthritis. The Glowbie crate is the first product designed to provide red light therapy to pets so that owners can treat their pets in the comfort of their own homes. For many reasons mentioned here, RLT is more acceptable than lasers. Lasers treatments would also cost more. Glowbies are, however, expensive for most pet owners. Note that it is possible to 'mock up' a cage or pet restraining area with a red light panel to get started at a lower cost. Fortunately for me, my dogs love the human pod "Med Bed" treatment; they relax in it, often with me, and they patiently wait for it to shut off automatically.

Chapter 5: RLT for Kids

Red light therapy (RLT), an encompassing term that includes visible red and near infra-red (NIR) light, is a safe and successful treatment for many pediatric conditions. RLT treats various ailments common in children, such as pain and neurological abnormalities.

One of the essential benefits that RLT may provide for children is that it does not cause any discomfort or perceived threat, so it isn't 'scary'. Unlike medications, side effects are extremely unlikely with RLT. RLT does not require making incisions or administering injections, making it a less intimidating alternative for children, including those who understandably fear needles or invasive, surgical procedures.

RLT is beneficial in treating several common skin conditions in children, such as eczema, acne, and diaper rash. These conditions can be very uncomfortable for children. RLT enhances skin texture and reduces inflammation just as it does for adults, alleviating itching and many other painful conditions. Typical healing is a relief to kids as symptoms decline with less stress. The severity and anxiety is more easily alleviated. This is particularly helpful for burns.

RLT has also been used to treat children who are afflicted with conditions such as juvenile arthritis and fibromyalgia. RLT lessens the discomfort that these conditions cause. By now there have been many studies that show RLT effectively reduces discomfort and inflammation, thereby improving the quality of life for children.

RLT shows promise as an option for youngsters afflicted with neurological diseases such as cerebral palsy and autism. Clinical trials have demonstrated that RLT improves muscle tone and reduces stiffness in children with cerebral palsy. RLT can bring about a beneficial outcome by improving the behavior and social connection of autistic children with others.

It's wise to seek out a skilled medical practitioner or pediatrician with sufficient RLT experience to prescribe an effective RLT protocol. Personalizing the treatment according to the specific needs of the child is essential for its effectiveness.

While RLT is generally considered safe for children, parents should take certain precautions before exposing them to it. Adults should discuss the possibility of protective eyewear if applicable or more comfortable. Medical advice suggests that children with specific health conditions (such as seizures) or those taking medication should consult their primary care physician before undergoing RLT.

RLT in Ophthalmology

Axial lengthening is a crucial factor in myopia, and it can increase the risk of future retinal disorders such as macular hemorrhage, glaucoma, retinal detachment or cataracts. Myopia is a refractive error that occurs when the eye becomes excessively elongated in the axial direction, causing the focal point to fall in front of the retina instead of directly on it. Ongoing research is currently investigating potential treatments aimed at slowing down the process of axial lengthening, which has been a longstanding concern. Examples of such treatments include modest doses of atropine drops and increasing outdoor time.

Potential Treatment for Autism

When using an infrared sauna with or without a red light therapy bed, a person with autism and a person who does not have autism should not experience any difference in how they use RLT. If a child has a chronic health problem then it is important to gradually increase the amount of time spent exposed to RLT. It is equally important to keep track of how the patient feels during and after a session. If you do this, you can gauge how well the RLT is helping the condition and monitor the child's anxiety..

Improved Well-Being & Stress Relief

One of the defining symptoms of autism is an elevated risk of experiencing anxiety and related disorders. Fortunately, several findings suggest that exposure to various parts of the red and infrared light spectrum can reduce anxiety. This approach is also crucial when addressing depression.

People who have autism may find that using RLT helps them alleviate symptoms of depression and anxiety. Reducing tension and anxiety levels is beneficial to kids and their parents.

Restful Sleep for Kids

Extensive evidence supports the effectiveness of red light therapy in promoting restful sleep in children of all ages, including toddlers, infants, and teenagers. Let's lay out the case for giving children red light therapy to help them sleep better every night.

Red Light versus Complete Darkness

Many parents worry that exposing their infants or toddlers to any light source in their bedroom may disrupt their ability to fall or stay asleep. Exposure to red light, instead of complete darkness, has measurable differences. Some believe newborns should be kept in total darkness because they have recently emerged from the dark environment of the mother's womb.

Even at 4-6 months, when sleep regression occurs, a fully dark environment can provoke fear and stress in babies and young children because their sleeping habits change as they mature over their first year. Children cannot comprehend the world around them if they wake up in the middle of the night in the dark. Using red light from the beginning creates a more calming and inviting environment for young children and it alleviates the issues associated with total darkness.

When parents switch on the red light for the first time in their child's room, they often worry that their children may experience difficulty falling asleep or staying asleep. This concern is prevalent among parents. In the first few days, the typical rhythm of sleeping may be disrupted or made worse; this may result in an increased amount of daytime sleepiness. Within a few days of RLT initiation in children, there is a positive effect on melatonin release from the pineal gland in the brain. The calming red light is very likely to have a calming influence on a child's disposition, and it will likely enhance their ability to fall asleep and remain asleep throughout the night.

Nightmares

Children are susceptible to nightmares. This anxiousness can involve being scared of the dark or believing that evil lurks in the shadows, or under the bed. Nightmares can cause children to act in inappropriate ways for their age. Children may also behave abnormally during the day after having nightmares. Putting your child to sleep using a television or iPad is not a good idea. Instead, consider getting your child a nightlight that emits red light. Children thrive with a set schedule, and receiving red light therapy helps establish a soothing, calm, and familiar environment.

Arranging your child's bedroom to simulate the beginning of twilight may encourage the human body to produce more melatonin. You may invest a few dollars in some blackout curtains or blinds to cover the windows and add a red night light to produce a pleasant glow in the room. This allows the child to fall asleep in an environment that simulates the sunset.

Conclusion

For a wide range of pediatric conditions, one treatment option that is virtually risk-free while highly effective is red light therapy. RLT treats various ailments common in children, such as pain and neurological abnormalities, and skin conditions. While administering the therapy to a child, it is advisable to follow the directions provided by a healthcare expert or an appropriate doctor. This will ensure the best possible outcome. Red light therapy can efficiently enhance childrens' general health and well-being when administered appropriately.

The findings powerfully demonstrate that light therapy not only leads to a significant and clinically meaningful improvement in behaviors associated with autistm in children and adolescents, it also shows progressive and meaningful symptom improvement for up to 6 months after completing the treatment. Similarly, RLT can produce significant improvement in general well-being for children and young adults without the risk of negative side-effects.

Chapter 6: RLT for Celebrities & Athletes

It's hard not to be amazed by how celebrities maintain such flawless skin. Look no further for the newest secret. It is no longer a mystery, and some celebrities, such as Jessica Alba, the Kardashian sisters, Kate Hudson, and many more, have even boasted about it on social networking sites.

Celebrities frequently test new anti-aging treatments before the public gains widespread access to them. Botox and other chemically induced anti-aging procedures, such as chemical face peels and injections of tissue fillers have been popular among Hollywood's A-listers for many years. On the other hand, Hollywood is moving away from harsh treatments, favoring the popularity of natural and holistic beauty trends of the past several years. In recent years, many A-list celebrities have consciously decided to avoid invasive surgical procedures in favor of more natural alternatives.

Celebrities increasingly turn to red light therapy, a natural and non-invasive anti-aging treatment, to look their best on screen and at red-carpet events. Kourtney Kardashian was relatively early to the scene in 2016 when she released a photo of herself wearing a red-light mask and touting the many anti-aging benefits of RLT. Since then, several other well-known celebrities, including Jennifer Lopez, Hillary Duff and Mandy Moore have spoken publicly about the beneficial effects that red and blue light facial therapy treatments have had on them.

Because of their devotion to RLT, many actors and actresses keep their own equipment in their homes. When asked about her facial routine in 2018, Olivia Munn told *US* magazine, "I have my own facial set up, I've got the professional-grade products and machines...But one of the best things is the red and blue light mask."

Red light therapy is effective because it boosts circulation and oxygen levels, providing the body's cells with the energy required to perform their functions more efficiently than in their own natural state. This technique helps to reduce inflammation and boost collagen formation, both of which diminish the appearance of fine lines and wrinkles, for smoother, firmer, more supple skin.

Designer of jewelry and reality television Star, Kristin Cavallari revealed to *Us Weekly* that she does not have Botox injections. She did, however, reveal in that interview, that "Red light treatment is something I do twice a week in order to keep fine lines and wrinkles at bay."

Red light therapy offers treatment possibilities beyond wrinkles and fine lines. With increasing popularity among celebrities, it's spreading from facial treatments over their entire bodies. Why? Using red light therapy devices, you can treat inflammation, joint pain and muscle soreness at home. The number of well-known people who advocate for red light treatment grows daily. Joan Smalls and Bella Hadid have visited celebrity aesthetician Joanna Czech's office regularly. Joanna Czech is well-known for the light treatments that she provides for her clients. Riverdale's Camila Mendes and Lili Reinhart have posted photographs from Joanna Vargas' red light bed on their Instagram accounts. This treatment is growing among the celebrity crowd, which often foreshadows acceptance for the general public. In this way, actors become the 'guinea pigs' for the rest of us!

It is becoming abundantly clear that the verdict is in: celebrities love red light therapy and its many benefits, both externally and internally. They have a growing experience with it to support all of the scientific research that shows it to be safe. If you desire a safe and more natural health and beauty treatment, then it’s no longer necessary to have superstar status! Everyone can enjoy the benefits of red-light therapy. You can experience these benefits right now in a spa, or in the convenience of your own home.

Anti-aging is a billion dollar industry. In Hollywood, the concept of aging is frowned upon and age is often the cause of celebrity insecurity. Thankfully, red light therapy can be safely used as an anti-aging treatment at home. Utilizing red light treatment equipment, we can all attain a red-carpet glow without the boutique prices celebrities are known to pay.

Fortunately, celebrities who have taken RLT treatment for a long time, both in-office and at home, have shared some of their experiences and divulged the benefits, and there is a substantial amount of research to back up their claims. Scientific research and this day-to-day experience act in concert to support an increasingly irrefutable belief in this therapy.

Kourtney Kardashian, an influencer in the fields of beauty and wellness, shared a throwback photo of herself on Instagram in 2016 wearing a luminous RLT mask, taken while she was at an appointment with famous aesthetician Shani Darden. Since Kardashian shared that pic, plenty of other stars, including Kelly Rowland, Chrissy Teigen, Emma Stone, Lena Dunham, and Real Housewives of New York City's Carole Radziwill, have posted images of themselves in similar red and blue light facial therapy sessions.

Since Kardashian and Alba published their first photos, the market has produced many LED light therapy devices designed for home use, available in a wide range of price points. According to Cherie Callahan, an Arizona-based aesthetician who has long employed LEDs in her practice, red light treatment penetrates the skin. It works by "increasing oxygen and blood flow," calling this "The food of cells." This speeds up biologic processes such as cell turnover, helping to decrease inflammation and enhancing collagen formation. Callahan told *Us Magazine* that she has used LEDs in her practice for a long time. She added, "Her skin is more supple with fewer fine lines and wrinkles because of using this treatment."

Technology has evolved beyond face masks to include hand-held devices and panels that can be hung on the wall, which means that you can now direct the light to other parts of your body to cure inflammation, joint pain, and muscle aches. Whole body pods are also on the rise among those who can afford the higher price tag, ranging around $80,000 and up!

Many professional athletes have publicly proclaimed that red light and near-infrared light therapy have operated in a synergistic manner to help them perform. Ara Suppiah, M.D., Founder of the Functional Sports Medicine Institute works with major champions like Phil Mickleson and Bubba Watson. Suppiah is also a true believer and outspoken supporter of RLT for sports injury recovery. According to *Us Weekly*, Ara Suppiah, M.D., one of the world's trusted medical pioneers in professional sports explains, "Increased energy within a muscle cell allows it to contract harder and repair itself better after training." The Institute is instrumental in finding ways for athletes to manage inflammation. It is evident that red light increases cellular energy production; it consequently helps organs, joints, and muscles repair themselves and function more optimally. Valerie Krossin of Aspen Laser also told me in 2023 that RLT has reduced training recovery time to 12 hours or less, enabling better performance for athletes. Aspen’s subsidiary, Theralight supplies RLT beds to at least 16 professional sports teams.

RLT supports the cells and the organs of the body, whether human or other animal, to perform with more energy, for longer times, and with enhanced recovery. While most at-home devices offer support or a modest boost of red light exposure between more intense sessions, more powerful in-office treatments are often more effective. Not everyone can afford to put large, professional RLT devices in their homes, but by combining affordable, at-home treatments with more complete and intense professional sessions, the general public can certainly enjoy some of the benefits of this therapy.

While filming *Infinite Power Workout* in the late 1990s, I had many famous guests who embodied extraordinary physiques. I was 30 to 33 years old and got a good look into true human potential. Some bodies are built with money in an operating room, and some are built with sweat and hard work in a gym. One of my dear guests was Dr. Garth Fisher, a world-famous plastic surgeon. That was around the time when the TV show *Doctor 90210* began its long run, based on Fisher' s work and his surgical cases. Dr. Fisher shared many pearls of wisdom with me over the years, but unlike red light therapy, plastic surgery always has a potential risk attached to it. I don't want to discount that *everything in life has some risk*. Still, when I would ask what he thought about me undergoing a particular surgical procedure, he would say to me, "Cie, if you were sitting at a Blackjack table and you had a 19, would you take a hit?" This was his way of saying that the risk was measurably greater than the potential reward. It was his creative way of talking me OUT of various cosmetic surgeries. I wish he had thought that I was holding a 20, but I'll be satisfied with the 19, and you get the idea. Instead of surgery, with its associated risk, Red Light Therapy is an easier decision. It doesn't have the same risks as surgery, so it's easier to accept as a universal antidote for aging, while promoting health and healing. We don't hear about the adverse side effects of red and near infra-red light therapy like we do a terrible facelift. There are no such 'horror stories'.

Noteworthy RLT Users

Clemson Tigers

Before winning the national championship, Clemson University added red light therapy (RLT) to its roster. In 2018 they established the Clemson Applied Science Lab at the Clemson University football facility. It came with two infrared hyper-thermic cocoon pods for far-infrared heat therapy to stimulate tissue regeneration and wound healing on a cellular level. That therapy was known to improve circulation and enhance cellular detoxification. Compression treatment machines, human contact massage chairs, and sensory deprivation pods are other rehabilitation technologies that Clemson University installed in its facilities. During that season, the Tigers had a perfect record, winning every game they played, including the national championship game against Alabama, with a final score of 44-16. Was it all attributable to RLT? Not 100% but considering the physical and mental components of treatment, critical thinking would truthfully affirm RLT’s substantial contribution to success.

Navy Seals

Members of the Navy SEAL team have used red light treatment since the 1990s to assist in the regeneration of muscle tissue and maintain their ranks' ability to function at high levels. After using red light therapy, members of the SEAL team experienced a reduction of more than 40 percent in the number of musculoskeletal training injuries while also experiencing a reduction in the amount of time it took for wounds to heal. Combining red light therapy with hyperbaric oxygen therapy was also observed to yield synergistic results. This is a combination also prescribed at Cerulean Human Health Performance for elite, competing athletes, as well as the rich and famous that visit the clinic in Phoenix from around the world.

Texas Rangers' Rehabilitation Process

Along with preventing and treating injuries, the medical team of the Texas Rangers works on rehabilitating baseball players so that they can return to the field at their highest possible level of performance. Red light therapy is a part of the Rangers' rehabilitation process, and the players entirely embrace and trust it. The Rangers' Sports Science department is responsible for implementing this therapy as part of the training process.

RLT for Improved Athletic Performance

When athletes encounter a novel or unfamiliar form of therapy, one of the most obvious questions they may ask is, "Will it enhance my performance or aid in my recovery?" The prognosis for red light therapy is favorable. However, the evidence is not entirely conclusive. Research has demonstrated some exciting benefits in enhancing athletic performance, including significant strength and endurance enhancements compared to a control group, and increased fatigue resistance during a maximal repetition test when applied during resting intervals. The next natural question for an athlete is, "When is the optimal time to use red and infrared light to get the most out of it?" Applying red and infrared light before strength training resulted in more significant strength increases. When endurance athletes received light therapy before *and* after training, their capacity for long-distance activity was enhanced threefold! Before beginning a workout, it is recommended to undergo a red light therapy session if increasing strength during the activity is the primary objective. Again, athletes who compete in endurance events appear to benefit the most from using red light before *and* after their workouts.

The red light bed at MVMT Fitness Club in Scottsdale, Arizona has a maximum time allowance of twenty minutes; beyond this point, the benefits begin to diminish significantly. Twenty minutes appears to be an accepted maximum treatment time for high radiance units that are scrutinized by champions, capable of developing a powerful recovery protocol, such as the owners at MVMT. Beyond this, if you move closer to the source of the red light, the light penetrates more effectively into the tissue, and the amount of time necessary to experience its therapeutic effects decreases. This is explained by the Inverse Law of Light or Inverse-Square Law; you can hear this explanation on my YouTube channel as explained by Ron Poe, the CEO and Founder of Red Light Wellness. You will find loads of information on RLT there and on my Muscle and Fitness+ TV channel.

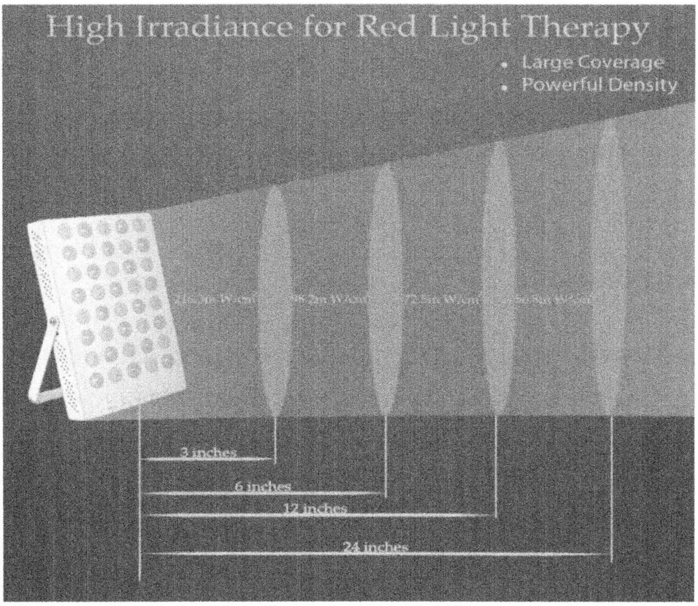

Tissue Recovery with RLT

The effects of infrared and red light for tissue recovery are not entirely consistent. The discomfort of soreness and inflammation resulting from injury to muscle tissue as a result of exercise is known as Delayed Onset Muscular Soreness (DOMS). Even though DOMS doesn't typically last for more than a few days after training, it can still lead to performance decreases when it is present. Because of this, during the in-season portion of training, coaches often program weight room sessions with decreased frequency and intensity to prevent negatively compromising the performance of their athletes during competition. Applying light therapy before an *eccentric* exercise routine helped to mitigate the detrimental effects of muscular injury and function from that session. It is important to note here that *eccentric* exercise is known to result in the most DOMS reaction compared to other workout routines, so it stands to reason that a modality to reduce such soreness would match well with it. Well-educated authorities in the world of RLT swear by it.

Conclusion

A well-researched therapeutic modality, red and infrared light has been shown to have a variety of positive effects on athletes without negative side effects. Athletes can see benefits in their sleep, their performance, and their soft tissue healing capacity when they adopt smart recovery strategies, including RLT. Of course, there is always a need for additional research to be done to support our conclusions. More will come in time, but with what we already know to be true, we may draw the conclusion that when red light therapy is used appropriately, it can lead to substantial athletic gains in a shorter amount of time than with training alone. The use of RLT before training is known to enhance strength and endurance, and treatment after training and competition has been proven to hasten recovery.

Chapter 7: How to Get Started with RLT

If you read the proceeding chapters, you know that there have been "happy experiments" with RLT. Frankly, this continues in 2023; we are *still* learning. The world has discovered that RLT, including NIR has the propensity to heal, beautify, regenerate and give us more quality years of life. This is exciting but there is much more to learn about effective and optimal RLT administration protocols. Responsible device companies are constantly testing their recommended protocols for users, while factories around the world manufacture their units, not fully understanding power, light radiance levels, and administrative protocols. This uncertainty may frighten some users. In all fairness, I have a medical disclaimer for a reason. I can tell you what research has shown, and what I would do, but I am a totally healthy 56 year old. I have had spectacular and wonderful results with a 4 wavelength bed, but when it comes to the small travel devices, I can't say they have yielded the results that I've hoped for. This is my personal experience combined with a higher-than-average understanding of the science.

I tried a small oral device that touts red and blue light. The blue is to whiten teeth and gel pens are also included in the kit. It stands to reason that healthier gums and whiter teeth are to be expected. I cannot say the standard protocol suggested by the device company is more effective than other treatments. I don't fear any negative side effects from using this device, so I may choose to continue with it, in a sense experimenting on myself, but so far I have not found it beneficial.

I've found that the real "bang for the buck" is using a commercial RLT bed for 4 to 5 days in a row. The first couple of days left me feeling no different, but after 4-5 days I absolutely knew that it worked. If the same protocol doesn't rock your world, then I would be very surprised. This is a more expensive route than many would accept. It is also more time-consuming to go into a facility regularly to use their equipment, which is why rich and famous people buy one to use at home. If this is an option you can save time, and over months and years you will also save money on sessions. Health professionals that have a clearer understanding of the benefits of RLT find it to be a good investment. Frankly, after the skin damage that I have done to myself in my youth with tanning beds, I hope to see tanning salons convert to RLT "Health" salons. They can start by using only half their space for RLT and giving clients a choice between tanning and RLT, prefaced with an education. This is a wave that could take hold and transform society in a healthy way. This is my beautiful vision for RLT spas everywhere.

I have given RLT masks to friends and business partners and they have touted some great results. Some say friends have actually complimented them for looking younger.

Charles Vorwaller, CEO of Aspen Laser/Theralight in Utah tells me, the reason that Theralight hasn't released a mask yet in such a hot market is because the delivery of even power across the surface depends on the physical contour of the mask. The CEO calls this homogeneous light output. If you are ready now, go ahead and choose a currently available unit if you can afford the price tag. I'm sure that given time, a company with decades of laser and RLT experience like Aspen Laser/Theralight will deliver an outstanding facial mask product that you can trust, but not until it's ready for primetime, and it may be under a different brand name. I will certainly update everyone through my own social media as such units are released to the public. There are also companies currently experimenting with bio-active topical products to boost RLT efficacy. I easily foresee an effective mask, combined with an amplifying topical agent, at an attainable price in the very near future!

If you decide to buy devices, I must say, let the buyer beware. Look for return policies, warranties, and don't buy products that are too weak. PBM is intended to be evidence-based. Devices are being rushed out of factories and many are made cheaply. Don't go with the cheapest if you are looking foer results. All devices are NOT created equal! Many manufacturers claim deeper penetration than what is delivered!

Light is energy. The healing provided by it is dependent on the dose, duration, and size of the area treated. Efficacy hasn't been proven for most available devices and it's not unusual for companies to skip this step. Low power and extended distances from red and NIR light are to be avoided. Low power is not to be confused with lower wavelengths that do red light or Low Level Laser Therapy; I am speaking about over-promising and under-delivering, which is common in this new science. You cannot be certain that higher radiance will deliver a better outcome. Data derived from trials and testing help the consumer to choose well. Try your device using the manufacturer' s protocols and if you are not getting results in 30 days, you have my permission to return it. Let the buyer beware.

My whole life is a search for the truth. If I see beds and devices that I would recommend, then they will be on my website and social media pages. I strive for true health and happiness for myself, and I believe that you deserve the same if you are willing to make the effort.

Regarding the canine market, if your pet allows it, then use your devices for them too if you choose not to incur the expense of a separate RLT crate. The devices work similarly whether they were designed for human or veterinary use. You may crawl into a canine crate, and you may put your dog in your RLT bed. You may find that both cats and dogs enjoy and benefit from the light just as you do, and this is worth a try. Ask your Vet if your pet is a candidate or has health concerns that may be problematic for RLT, but this is unlikely. Don't overdo it, and monitor results as you would for yourself. Jolie, my alpha dog started with a small travel device and enjoyed it. Now she is the first to jump into my commercial bed every morning. Although I don't own a horse and I don't ever plan to, I have checked out the line of products at RLTvet.com; they have tested many products for the equine market. I will share more on social media and my website when I feel strongly that new products are beneficial.

With all of this said, RLT may not be for everyone. I certainly believe it is for most! There is a current attitude of "point and shoot" as if PBM is as simple as a digital camera. Although this isn't scientific, it may work for most of us, or at least it will do no harm. Unfortunately, as a writer I cannot know your specific needs or concerns, I haven't seen your labs; I don't know your health or family history and I don't know your chosen vices. I do hope to see you invest your time and resources into the best health that you can afford. These products and treatments probably won't be covered by your health insurance. Steer towards functional medicine and cellular health. If your doctor doesn't know these terms it may be time to get a new doctor. Many concierge practices have misinformed my personal friends regarding bio-identical hormones, wrongly prescribing them and having no idea about RLT. This is expensive poor guidance! I left my traditional OB-GYN 8 years ago for not having the knowledge to answer my questions about hormone supplementation, and I am very happy that I did. With this said, I am doing my own study with a statistical N of 1, that is proving to show me that RLT is complimenting my plant-based, bio-identical hormone treatments; this means I need less hormone dose for the same youthful result since I've added RLT. With labs taken regularly, you can see how much Total Testosterone and Estrogen you have, and I dare say, for women in their 40's, most women have just an insignificant trace. It's no wonder we feel groggy, brain-fogged, and we don't have the energy to go to the gym. We struggle with our weight and our libido. Check my social media sources for more information regarding this- it all flows into a comprehensive anti-aging program.

Final Thoughts

It's evident that red light therapy is a viable alternative to toxic or unhealthy "health programs." RLT continues to gain popularity. These standard and alternative modalities need to be integrated, as both have their roles for our health maintenance. RLT's non-invasive and non-toxic nature and its potential to safely promote numerous health benefits have led to its widespread acceptance in many healthcare settings and salons. As research brings us closer to calculating optimal administration, we will see it used to treat more life-threatening and debilitating diseases in concert with allopathic and osteopathic approaches. This integrated vision is very close on the horizon.

Throughout this book, we explored the science behind red light therapy along with its history and application. We now understand how red light therapy works, including its capacity to boost mitochondrial function and the promotion of cellular repair and regeneration.

We've also discussed the possible benefits of red light treatment for various ailments, such as skin disorders, pain management, wound healing, and promotion of mental health. Having read this book we now understand and appreciate that inflammation is a normal part of the workings of the body and the immune system, but excessive inflammation is the origin of most physical diseases. We now understand that the primary benefit of RLT is modulation of inflammation, so it can prevent it from growing out of control. We've looked at the mounting body of evidence supporting RLT's use in preventing and treating many chronic diseases like SAD, Autism, diabetes, wound healing, and even cancer.

Even though more research is needed to fully understand the mechanism of red light therapy's action, and its potential applications in health promotion, the evidence thus far is compelling. As technology advances, red light therapy is destined to become a more accepted and accessible therapy for a myriad of health issues.

Overall, this book has offered a thorough overview of red light treatment, emphasizing its numerous potential benefits and explaining its importance in alternative, functional, and integrative medicine. This book is an essential resource for understanding the science and applications of red light therapy, whether you are a researcher, a healthcare professional, or simply a consumer interested in researching alternative remedies for your family and your pets.

As America's #1 Body, Mind and Spirit expert in my younger years, and now a longevity expert 25 years later, it is my aim to continue shining 'light' on the best information possible for my audience so they may experience the healthiest outcomes possible. Some of the finest and latest data can be found in PubMed. You can find PubMed online and fact-check information for yourself. It is the National

Library of Medicine from the National Institute of Health. It can be a little daunting for those who are not trained in the medical field; there is a lot of jargon and science that might not be readily understandable. Please know that I am committed to deciphering this information for you and sharing it with you in words that non-medical people can appreciate and understand. Please check my YouTube regularly for additional practical wisdom. My channel can be found under Cie Allman-Scott or @cieallmanscott, and my website and Instagram are DoctorCie.com and @DoctorCie. I also post on Facebook. I will share new information from the actual researchers in this book and the device manufacturers discussed here as it becomes available.

My purpose is to provide empowerment for the unlimited possibilities for all people, including that which is optimal for the development of the body, mind, and Spirit. My mission hasn't changed in 30 years. Please know it to be enduring, as is my commitment to you, my audience. I will remain diligent yet humble in sharing the truth. I never quit, and I still have the strength to do it. I share all of my secrets. Please check out my work, be inspired, and reach your highest potential. This is what I wish for you.

About The Author

Cie Allman-Scott, Ph.D. is a seasoned show host and Media Psychologist who successfully evolved to both sides of the camera. During the years hosting her first episodic daily talk show, Dr. Cie was frequently asked to write for health and fitness magazines. She was a featured celebrity writer for many, contributing monthly columns for publications like Max Muscle and Fitness. After the demands of a daily TV series ended, she wrote her first book, *7 Rules for Making Decisions* and developed many timeless tools for self-help, including many audio books and self development programs. Dr. Cie continues with *over 20* years lecturing throughout the world, usually keynoting brain optimization topics. Dr. Cie is also the writer of TV commercials, infomercials, episodic and "how to" daytime TV programs. Dr. Cie has over thirty years of full time experience as an actress, TV host and narrator, including voice-overs for hundreds of productions. Having an executive hand in many programs and long ago specializing in Direct Response advertising, she uses her degree in Psychology to influence and inspire television viewers to think intensely and to be healthy and fit. With experience as a powerful teacher, her career in modeling, acting, and hosting afforded her a unique education, which included improvisation and comedy. She played prankster parts on Totally Hidden Video, Saturday Night Live, and also performed stand-up comedy at The Improv in L. A. Cie understands the value of a comedic edge and uses humor divinely in hundreds of celebrity interviews for FOX, ABC, CBS, and UPN television. Feeling creatively incomplete reading lines for recurring roles on General Hospital, Baywatch, and many other episodics, her self expression took over and she created *Infinite Power Workout*, a daytime, celebrity-driven TV show which she grew from 3 markets to 186 on major networks. Executive Producing her show afforded her the opportunity to learn most TV production jobs and successfully syndicate her own show. Focused on her tasks, she became an excellent writer; advertising clients were also pleased with her ability to research and execute meaningful scripts. As the owner of a production company, she also produced commercials for large, world-wide companies such as LifeFitness, Toto, and Stevia. She produced martial arts videos, exercise videos, as well as TV series and films, such as *Idol Chat* with the all-star casts Dr. Cie watched as a child including *Love Boat, Happy Days* and *E.T.* Dr. Cie Scott now cherry picks TV and film projects, writes inspiring self-help books, blogs and creates content, and is a voting member of the Academy of Television Arts and Sciences. She is also a member of both SAG and AFTRA. As an actress, TV host and producer, "Dr. Cie" earned 9 Tellys, 2 Vision Awards, and 2 Primetime Emmy nominations for production and hosting. Current projects include producing, writing and hosting *Beauty and Truth* and *Longevity Reports with Dr. Cie*, distributed world-wide on over 100 known TV apps like Amazon, Apple TV and Muscle and Fitness+.

In 2019 she wrote the Amazon #1 best-seller, *DECIDE YOUR FUTURE; Write, Direct and Star in Your Life*. This book is helpful for any person and allows life to be an "open book test" rather than a series of frustrations. Dr. Cie is tirelessly driven to inform and inspire audiences to make life all it can be. "Suffering is optional!" and "Life is what YOU make it!" are regular quotes she will repeat until audiences understand, believe and achieve their personal goals.

Dr. Cie is a passionate world traveler and a member of the Travelers Center Club, having visited 158 countries to date. Cie loves to scuba dive, dance and discover food, wine and chocolate. She lives with her husband, retired General and

Dr. Cie Allman-Scott

Vascular Surgeon, Aaron Scott and their therapy dogs, Papillons, Jewell, Jolie, and future AKC show dogs, Angelique and Estee.

Links and Resources

https://doctorcie.com/

https://www.youtube.com/c/cieallmanscott

https://www.instagram.com/doctorcie/

https://www.facebook.com/DrCie/

https://www.imdb.com/name/nm0021515/

https://twitter.com/jetsetphd

https://www.linkedin.com/in/cie/

https://www.amazon.com/stores/author/B07QQVKNQD

http://www.jetsetphd.com/ Travel like a Pro!

INDEX

I

K

L

M

N

O

P

R

S

T

V

W

Also by Cie Allman-Scott, Ph. D.

DECIDE YOUR FUTURE; Write, Direct and Star in Your Life

(Paperback, Kindle) ISBN 10: 0-9774811-1-

5 ISBN 13: 97809774811-5-6) 2019

Now LIFE is an "open book test." Choose your path. Use the personalized 7 steps for making decisions and succeed at every goal.

Recognize and overcome the glitches in the human mind that are misguiding you. Find certainty, clarity and confidence.

Live free and purposefully. Use a combination of your desires, your intuition and new skills to succeed and create the life you have always wanted.

THE PEOPLE MAGNET

(CD Audio book) ISBN 10: 0-9774811-1-

5 ISBN 13: 978097748118) 2009

Listen Today! Attract Immediately! Flip the switch to success!

Realize 21 keys to relate better to others, and enjoy a better connection with all people when you 'remove the static.'

If you're coming up short in life---no committed partner, no great clients, or maybe you just want to attract people to date, or to nail a good job---you may need a People Magnet! You can release and extend your magnetic power! This audio book will improve your relationships, finances, and health! Attract in every trajectory, energizing the Law of Attraction; you will easily comprehend 21 principled strategies or simple changes you can implement immediately to remove barriers and connect to others! You will also instantly enjoy a happier and more confident demeanor. You can stop repelling people, money, and vitally important health! Unblock your true Infinite Power today with THE PEOPLE MAGNET!

REINVENT YOURSELF

(CD Audio book/ Audio Download)

ISBN: 9780966225730

Earn big money without competition by doing what you love!

Finding your purpose aligns you with doing what you love and getting paid! Enjoy easy and fun exercises to find your purpose and happiness in under 30 minutes! Use this passion to create your dream job! As you work for yourself, you forge a career that resonates with you and your genuine inner enthusiasm! Affirmations and guided meditation tracks reduce fear and empower every user; these tracks can be used every day! This product facilitates instant clarity and confidence, self respect, self-awareness, and breakthroughs! The process is easy to do anywhere and can be effective every time in your life you need to progress with paradigm shifts, and reinvent yourself again.

THE GODDESS CODE: Your Secret Weapon for Dating Success!

ISBN 13: 978-0-94811-4-9 (Audio download)

The Goddess Code is the single girls' therapy and guidance for successful dating, straight from the host of The Goddess Code, on iTunes, Stitcher.com, YouTube and Facebook Live! You can establish trust and commitment with a KEEPER and FORGET the losers forever! IT is 100% effective for repairing your self esteem and putting you on the correct path to find the one you desire. The Goddess Code works for young and old. It works for all genders. Dr. Cie Scott interviewed

over 20,000 singles coast to coast, who were seeking "THE ONE." These men and women provided the groundwork for the keys to find commitment in a world of serial monogamy, pain, and disrespect! Find timeless, perfect answers immediately and useful keys to create the life you want to live and the path to your loving partner! These keys to commitment are EXPLICIT and CRYSTAL CLEAR, so implementing them immediately creates instant dating success and order in your life. Want to know if someone is truthful with you? Never put your self respect on the line and never lose control again! Get started today! Gain the confidence and clarity you need to find a winner in a sea of undesirable partners. Reduce your stress level and stop struggling with THE GODDESS CODE; it's your secret weapon! Stop your harmful patterns today! This special release goes beyond the podcast and free information, and if you are finished making mistakes, you can't afford to skip over it!

Dr. Cie Allman-Scott

MEDITATION FOR BEGINNERS and INTERMEDIATE:
Natural Stress Release, Anti-Aging and Self Realization

(CD Audio book/Audio Download) ISBN: 978-0-977481132

Guided Meditations and easy instruction allow you to meditate and overcome previous obstacles in this simple, pleasurable process. Deep relaxation techniques allow you to rejuvenate for better overall health, and clarity results from this daily meditation habit! Instant gratification:

- Tranquility and Unshakable Confidence
- Creative Solutions & Clarity of Mind
- Increased Energy and Better Health
- Discover Daily Peace
- Improve Your Relationships & Finances

POWERFUL DAILY AFFIRMATIONS FOR SUCCESS

(CD/ Audio Download)

Listen daily for transformation, inspiration and unshakable confidence! Relax, listen and repeat after Dr. Cie! You can reprogram the negativity you have collected over time and find a confident outlook on life that lasts and alters your future for the better.

You can find most audio downloads at TheAudioBookMarket.com and check my "Tool Box" (online store) at DoctorCie.com

Made in the USA
Monee, IL
10 April 2025

15546679R00066